Reimagining Disabli:
Violence as Abjectio

MW01579193

Drawing upon vivid and harrowing life history narratives of people labelled intellectually disabled, this book examines the ways in which disabled subjects are constituted, regulated, governed, and violated through an account of abjection.

Extending interdisciplinary dialogues and approaches, it abandons a construct of violence (which by law requires a stable notion of a victim and a perpetrator) and moves to a theorisation of abjection to explore the ways in which disabled subjects are (re)produced, constituted, and treated through time. Deploying a wide range of interdisciplinary approaches, this book sits at the intersections of criminology and sociology, re-thinks notions of dis/ ability, violence, and subjectivity, and utilises crip and queer theory to imagine dis/ability differently.

It will be of interest to all scholars and students of disability studies, sociology and criminology, and specifically those working in the areas of life history work, post-structuralism, hate crime, and post-modern criminology.

Ryan Thorneycroft is Lecturer in Criminology at Western Sydney University, Australia.

Interdisciplinary Disability Studies

Series editor:
Mark Sherry, *The University of Toledo, USA*

Disability studies has made great strides in exploring power and the body. This series extends the interdisciplinary dialogue between disability studies and other fields by asking how disability studies can influence a particular field. It will show how a deep engagement with disability studies changes our understanding of the following fields: sociology, literary studies, gender studies, bioethics, social work, law, education, or history. This ground-breaking series identifies both the practical and theoretical implications of such an interdisciplinary dialogue and challenges people in disability studies as well as other disciplinary fields to critically reflect on their professional praxis in terms of theory, practice, and methods.

Disability Hate Speech
Social, Cultural and Political Contexts
Edited by Mark Sherry, Terje Olsen, Janikke Solstad Vedeler and John Eriksen

Sexual Citizenship and Disability
Understanding Sexual Support in Policy, Practice and Theory
Julia Bahner

Critical Disability Studies and the Disabled Child
Unsettling Distinctions
Harriet Cooper

Disability, Globalization and Human Rights
Edited by Hisayo Katsui and Shuaib Chalklen

Reimagining Disablist and Ableist Violence as Abjection
Ryan Thorneycroft

Identity Construction and Illness Narratives in Persons with Disabilities
Chalotte Glintborg and Manuel de la Mata

Reimagining Disablist and Ableist Violence as Abjection

Ryan Thorneycroft

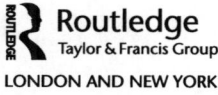

Routledge
Taylor & Francis Group

LONDON AND NEW YORK

First published 2020
by Routledge
2 Park Square, Milton Park, Abingdon, Oxon OX14 4RN

and by Routledge
52 Vanderbilt Avenue, New York, NY 10017

Routledge is an imprint of the Taylor & Francis Group, an informa business

British Library Cataloguing-in-Publication Data
A catalogue record for this book is available from the British Library

Library of Congress Cataloging-in-Publication Data
Names: Thorneycroft, Ryan, 1990- author.
Title: Reimagining disablist and ableist violence as abjection / Ryan
Thorneycroft.
Description: Abingdon, Oxon ; New York, NY : Routledge, 2020. |
Series: Interdisciplinary disability studies | Includes bibliographical
references and index.
Identifiers: LCCN 2020011171 (print) | LCCN 2020011172 (ebook) |
ISBN 9780367365547 (hbk) | ISBN 9780429347887 (ebk)
Subjects: LCSH: Discrimination against people with disabilities. |
People with disabilities–Crimes against. | Rejection (Psychology)
Classification: LCC HV6250.4.H35 T55 2020 (print) | LCC
HV6250.4.H35 (ebook) | DDC 305.9/08–dc23
LC record available at https://lccn.loc.gov/2020011171
LC ebook record available at https://lccn.loc.gov/2020011172

ISBN: 978-0-367-36554-7 (hbk)
ISBN: 978-0-429-34788-7 (ebk)

Typeset in Times
by Integra Software Services Pvt. Ltd.

Contents

Formatting and other conventions

This book presents unedited excerpts from the people who participated in the research upon which this book is based. The excerpts are presented in this way to maintain veracity to the ways in which the participants—and all of us—communicate verbally, including intonations, contradictions, false starts, stuttering, and so on. Specifically, I aim to illuminate the crip temporality with which the participants spoke.

Ellipses (…) are used in the narrative to indicate where material has been omitted.

The text in parentheses within the interview transcript excerpts is me, the interviewer, unless otherwise specified.

All of the names mentioned in this book are pseudonyms.

Preface

Much of the content for this book was written in 2016 and 2017 following interviews collected between May 2015 and April 2016 for my doctoral research conducted at the School of Social Sciences and Psychology at Western Sydney University. Once written, I have only turned back to the text sparingly—almost exclusively to find an odd reference that eluded me while writing other work. Over the past few months I have needed to return to this work to materialise it into the book you have before you. I confess it has been a struggle to look back on. The theoretical mistakes and omissions notwithstanding, I struggle to look back on this text because of the profoundly emotional experience this part of my life constituted. The stories contained within this book are emotional and heart-wrenching, and I still cannot shake them.

In 2014 I wanted to interview victims of disablist violence as part of my doctoral project. Originally I was interested in heterosexist violence, yet as I was closeted at the time, any inference of *being gay* needed to be repelled. I then thought of my disabled sister, Mahnie, and decided to focus my attention on disablist violence. At the time, the visibility of her disability seemed a safer alternative to the invisibility of my queerness. Since then, the ethics and politics of in/visibility have informed the development of my work, particularly with my theoretical focus on abjection.

Reflecting back, I wanted to get a sense for what violence *felt like* for disabled people. While I have experienced violence in my life, I wanted to understand it from their perspective. What I failed to comprehend was the ways in which I would be so affected by their stories, as well as my incessant reflections on the ethics, politics, and inherent violence of research. My focus on the theory of abjection also did not help me—I carry their stories and this abjection around like a brick. In reading the pages that unfold, I ask the reader to reflect on the politics of research. In modernist neo-liberal university settings, research often serves and benefits the researchers more than anyone else—in terms of employment, promotions, and prestige. As Goodley and Runswick-Cole (2012: 215) suggest, 'research is an imperialist, disablist and heteronormative peculiarity of modernist knowledge production'. Research might be understood as an inherently exploitative venture, where the principles of beneficence can never be ensured, potential harm can never be erased, and research can only ever be judged efficacious after, *not before*, its completion.

In any case, I send this research out and into the world. While it may help in the conversion of my university employment contract from fixed-term to ongoing (perhaps, boss?), I do it for another more important reason. It may seem ironic that I seek to spread stories that I have almost never re-read since first writing them, but I need to share them because I can no longer sit with them alone. Their stories haunt me, and I need to send them out. In a sense, I am taking in their abjection and I am asking the reader to take it up. Perhaps they will be able to take it, to use it, repackage it; perhaps even queer or crip it. If what I am writing to you now does not make much sense, never mind, it might by the time you have finished reading this book.

Much of what I wrote in my thesis has been copy and pasted into this book, except for the conventional evisceration of the 'Methods' chapter. This is a shame because in it I laboured over the politics of the research, my approaches to it, and the ableist and disablist tropes existent within research and its production. In any case, certain sacrifices—or norms—need(?) to be acquiesced. This means all the mistakes stay—and for that, I guess I apologise. This book, then, and the stories presented therein, should be contextualised by the intersections, experiences, and histories of doctoral work. Such work has time constraints, competing demands, precarity and precariousness, and the emerging skills of an early career researcher—and all of these traits are imprinted on the stories in this book in some way. Perhaps my submission of this book can be contextualised as an embracement of failure; as a performative politics that overwrites the logics of success and perfection.

Several people have played a profound role in helping me materialise the research idea into a piece of text. Particularly, I thank Nicole Asquith and Peter Bansel, who both helped me in their own unique ways. Lives are inherently complicated, stressful, and tough, and I thank you both for allowing me to enter your lives and take up your time while I have been on this journey. I also thank Fiona Kumari Campbell and Jen Slater, who both provided important critiques and feedback on my original doctoral thesis. Most of all, however, I want to thank the thirteen people who have contributed their lives and stories to this study. I am forever grateful, and your stories have moved me more than I ever imagined. I also thank the support workers who helped the participants; thank you for your support.

It's amazing how friendships come and go, or most often in my case, elude me completely. Hopefully one day I will get over my self-destructive tendencies. In any case, I would also like to thank Dan Perell, Laura Dunne, Justin Mahlberg, Dan Talbot, Ashley Talbot, and Jarrod Lambkin. Thank you. To my parents, my sister, and my brother—I love you all so much. And to Freddie—you're my rock.

In reading this text, I ask the reader for their patience and their perseverance. It is heavy-going. I cover dense theoretical ground and the participant's stories are harrowing. Take your time, and reach out to others if you need. Think about the ways in which abject lives experience abjection, but perhaps most importantly, try and think about the ways in which it can be resisted and/or reimagined.

Ryan Thorneycroft
February 2020
Sydney
Australia

Reference

Goodley, D and Runswick-Cole, K 2012, 'Decolonising Methodology: Disabled Children as Research Managers and Participant Ethnographers', in *Inclusive Communities: A Critical Reader*, edited by A Azzopardi and S Grech, Sense Publishers, Rotterdam, pp. 215–232.

1   Beginnings

Disabled bodies and subjects are ubiquitously constituted as 'other'. They are simultaneously everywhere and nowhere, over-victimised and under-recognised. In this book, I interrogate and reimagine disablist and ableist violence as abjection. I specifically resist the medicalisation and pathologisation of disabled bodies and lives, and work with an account of abjection as simultaneously psychic and social in order to articulate sites, practices, and possibilities for resistance. The basis for this account is built upon thirteen life history narratives I conducted with people labelled intellectually disabled in Australia in 2015–2016. My arrival to abjection was not a straightforward or linear process. In what follows, I give an account of the ways in which both the research topic and my position as researcher changed from inception to conclusion.

Originally a hate crime researcher within the field of criminology, I set out to research intellectually disabled people's experiences of disablist violence. Prior to and during the data collection periods, however, I developed several uncertainties with the topic that eventually impacted the project. These uncertainties emerged from both pragmatic issues such as methodological dilemmas, and the revision of my own theoretical trajectory. This ultimately led me to change the topic of my research. What was originally titled 'Disablist Violence, Victimisation and the Regulation of Prejudice' has become 'Reimagining Disablist and Ableist Violence as Abjection'. What was previously a structuralist account of hate crime experience with a criminological focus turned into a post-structuralist account of abjection, disability, and subjectivity within a critical disability studies framework. Below, I briefly document some of the aforementioned uncertainties that led to this shift in topic. I do this to position the book in a particular way, and to highlight to the reader that research, including my own, is never a linear journey from one point to another. Rather, research is messy, non-linear, and reiterative, and this is inherently the case when complex objects constitute the object of inquiry (Law 2004; Law and Singleton 2005).

A key uncertainty emerged from my ongoing and complicated relationship with the conceptual definition of hate crime. Definitions of hate crime have varied over time, though original conceptualisations took a literal approach to hate crime, meaning they were crimes motivated by hatred. While it has been increasingly recognised that hate crimes are motivated by bias and prejudice, I felt that there was an uneasy distance between my understanding of it and that of other hate crime scholars. For instance, in my thinking, hate crime did not require hatred or criminal conduct to be enacted; hate crime as I have come to understand it involves both physical and non-physical, legal and illegal practices against oppressed minorities. Hence, I became more interested in the micro-practices, or normative violence (Butler 1990, 2004), that oppress minority populations.

At a broader level, I was concerned with the politics of the hate crime movement. While it is certainly laudable that the victimisation of minorities is adequately punished, hate crime as a construct is tied to identity politics. According to Jacobs and Potter (1998: 13–14), identity politics refers to

> a politics whereby individuals relate to one another as members of competing groups based upon characteristics like race, gender, religion, and sexual orientation. According to the logic of identity politics, it is strategically advantageous to be recognized as disadvantaged and victimized. The greater a group's victimization, the stronger its moral claim on the larger society.

As inferred from this quote, there is a 'competition of suffering' (Mason-Bish 2013: 20) where each collective must lay claim for remedial action. Fraser (2003) suggests this does little to address the underlying structures that perpetuate oppression. Another flaw I perceived is the way in which identity and its politics are constructed. According to Crenshaw (1991: 1242), identity politics 'conflates or ignores intragroup differences', and it elides issues of class (Fraser 2003). More importantly, however, is that identity politics seems to presuppose that identities are fixed. This mobilised yet another uncertainty, leading me to question the extent to which identities are stable or fixed. As Butler (1990: 142) argues,

> [t]he foundationalist reasoning of identity politics tends to assume that an identity must first be in place in order for political interests to be elaborated and, subsequently, political action to be taken. My argument is that there need not be a 'doer behind the deed,' but that the 'doer' is variably constructed in and through the deed.

Identities, in Butler's (1990) account, are constructed, contestable, contingent, and performed, rather than fixed and natural. Further, Butler (1990: 148) argues that identity politics 'presumes, fixes, and constrains the very "subjects" that it hopes to represent and liberate'. My concern was/is that identity politics, in spite of its admirable cause, might work to re-instantiate the oppression that it paradoxically seeks to overcome.

Another uncertainty lay with my methodological approaches. As the objects of my inquiry were people labelled intellectually disabled and their experiences of hate crime, I needed to construct a method that would yield the sort of results I was setting out to achieve (that is, experiences of hate crime). As I was neither experienced nor particularly interested in using quantitative methods, it became clear that some sort of interviewing needed to occur. Instead of interviewing the parents, carers, or guardians of people labelled intellectually disabled—a disablist and ableist practice that is unfortunately too common—I wanted to privilege the stories of people labelled intellectually disabled. This presented a number of challenges: I did not want the interviews to be unnecessarily traumatic, and I recognised the range of possible communication barriers between disabled and abled people[1] inherent to ableist societies. I therefore decided to focus more broadly on the participants' life experiences as evoked through life history interviews, which Plummer (2001: 18) describes as an 'account of one person's life in his or her own words'. Inevitably, the participants' accounts of experience opened up possibilities and trajectories that I had not anticipated, and the topics under inquiry became increasingly broad. So, what was originally framed as 'experiences of hate crime' came to focus more generally on 'life experiences'.

Recruitment strategies posed further challenges. Unlike the United Kingdom or the United States, there is no Australian data pool (such as complaints to police)—public or private—that documents victims of disablist hate crime. This meant that alternative strategies for locating possible participants needed to be adopted, and I approached advocacy organisations to assist in the recruitment of participants who had experienced hate crime. I was originally intending to employ purposive sampling (experiences of hate crime), but as I listened to the participants' stories, I realised that the narrow framing of the interview was problematic. Some of the participants did not describe experiences that corresponded with hate crime, and this complicated the purpose and focus of my research. Moreover, while some of the participants narrated experiences that might be understood as acts of hate crime, they did not describe them in such terms. I therefore became increasingly reluctant to impose the construct of hate crime on their experiences, not only because they had not articulated it as such, but because I was becoming increasingly concerned with the field of hate crime itself.

During the stages of the research contained within this book I started to read queer theory for my own personal and political interest. This moved my thinking in significant ways. I became preoccupied with my own queer subjectivity, my own ab/normality, and my infuriation with normative standards. As Goodley (2014: 159) says—I think quite poetically—'normative standards have the potential to feed some pretty fucked up responses to that which is deemed to be abnormal'. These ideas bled into my research and this book, and I started to read critical disability studies.

Critical disability studies is a transdisciplinary, relativist, and post-conventionalist school of thought. It works to disrupt and critique conventional, normative, and essentialist understandings of disability, and to interpret the lived experiences of disability and constructions of dis/ability (see Campbell 2009a; Goodley 2013; McRuer 2002; Meekosha and Shuttleworth 2009; Shildrick 2009, 2012; Slater 2015). Dis/ability is a split term that denotes the ways in which ability and disability, ableism and disablism, are constituted in simultaneous relation to one another. Shildrick (2012: 37) suggests that critical disability studies is guided by the question of, 'what it would mean, ontologically and ethically, to reimagine dis/ability as the very condition of human becoming'. I came to situate my project within this critical disability studies framework, because it became apparent to me that my structuralist/criminological/violence/hate crime paradigm was no longer compatible with my emergent thinking about the politics of non/normative lives, and that it needed to be abandoned in favour of a new focus on abjection.

From violence to abjection

In accordance with life history work, the interview technique I adopted was semi-structured. It is tempting to say parts of interviews were unstructured, as on multiple occasions the interviews were flexible, went down any path chosen by the participant, and were minimally guided by myself. Yet it would be misleading to suggest that I went into any interview without thoughts, ideas, or issues that influenced the interaction. The initial focus of the interviews was on experiences of hate crime, but as they progressed, the experiences the participants articulated pushed me towards other interests and topics. I started to see patterns in the ways they were talking about their experiences and themselves, and these initiated shifts in my thinking towards questions of pathologisation, ab/normality, dis/ability, dis/avowal, and so on. Rather than direct my attention to experiences of violence (or hate crime), I was moved to contextualise the participants' experiences within broader discussions about prejudice, subjectivity, and normativity.

Violence, as a framing concept, became too reductive in my analysis, especially since by law, violence requires a perpetrator and a victim. My imperative became to abandon this paradigm and move from a construct of violence to a theorisation of abjection. I pursue abject/tion as a framing concept because it simultaneously incorporates and extends the notion of violence. As Tyler (2009: 87) writes, '[d]isgust reactions, hate speech, acts of physical violence and the dehumanizing effects of law are integral to processes of abjection'. The concept of abjection incorporates perpetration and victimisation at the same time as it blurs the boundaries between them (Kristeva 1982). Rather than use ableism as the central frame, I consider that ableism is actually structured by abjection (see Young 1990). By using abjection, I am able to explain (disablist and ableist) violence from multiple scales, sites, and perspectives (Tyler 2013). In this book I am using abjection to theorise disabled people's experiences of disablist and ableist violence, not as an objective and totalising account of their experiences, but as an intellectual tool that enables me to reconsider dominant narratives about disability that pervade the field.

Abjection, which etymologically means to 'cast out', refers to the conditions in which subjects are rendered unintelligible according to regulatory norms, and it has increasingly been used to comprehend the oppression of various minority groups (see McClintock 1995; Tyler 2013; Warin 2010; Young 1990, for example). To be clear, I am not substituting violence for abjection. I argue that abjection—in contrast to stable notions of violence—opens up greater spaces of possibility and agency. Technologies of abjection are not stable practices; rather, abjection is produced and reproduced, and shapes the subject over time. There are also spaces in, and practices through which, abjection can be resisted. Because abject/ion refers to a subject position that is socially constituted, moving from a construct of violence to a theorisation of abjection demands that I engage with notions of subjectivation so I can interrogate violence as abjection. In the next section, I consider three concepts central to this book: the (disabled) body, the disabled subject, and abjection.

The (disabled) body

A large body of research is based on and reproduces objectivist understandings of (intellectual) disability, and this is also reflected among broader societal beliefs. These perspectives assume the external reality of things; whereby naturalised ontological facts can be objectively observed through our senses to discover reality. This viewpoint assumes that meaning is universal, and exists within objects of inquiry. Objectivism lays claim to a 'reality' that can be broken down and observed through scientific and objective methods to produce 'knowledge' or 'truth'. Within the context of disability, impairment is presumed to be a natural biological fact, and this presumption is widespread in society (Oliver 1996). Notwithstanding other epistemological viewpoints (such as constructionism or realism), I subscribe to a subjectivist epistemology and presume that reality and knowledge are interpretive rather than value-free. Whereas objectivist epistemology posits that the object (of inquiry) exists independent of the subject, subjectivist epistemology argues that the object is only ever produced and made intelligible by the individual or collective subject. Subjectivists argue that meaning is imposed, created, or produced by the subject and placed upon the object. Pratt (1998: 24) summarises the subjectivist position thus:

> knowledge (and truth) is dependent upon what individuals bring to the moment of perception. Knowledge and truth are created, not discovered; the world is only knowable through people's interpretations of it ... knowledge is neither a copy nor a mirror of some external reality but, rather, a construction of the individual experiencing it. People (learners) do not merely respond to the world; they impose meaning and value upon it and interpret it in ways that fit, or make sense to them.

According to a subjectivist epistemology, knowledge is value-laden and created, and an awareness of this is central to the ways in which I engage with the embodiment of people labelled intellectually disabled in this book. As Galvin (2003: 84–85) illustrates,

> [w]hen someone is named 'disabled', they are not being accorded a tag that simply describes a physical and material condition, they are being ascribed a set of oppressive associations that stem from the hypostatisation of an abstract concept.

I argue that the meaning 'disability' does not come from an interaction between the subject and object, but is placed upon the object—by an individual or collective subject—to constitute (disabled) existence. While this interpretation might not seem to allow disabled people agency, throughout this book—and particularly in Chapter 2—I discuss disability as both an imposed and (re)claimed subjectivity. Particularly, I am interested in the doubleness of this subjectification and how the 'dis/abled' subject is constituted, and the possibility for the subject to resist and reclaim the term as one of pride.

In *Bodies that Matter* (1993), Butler argues that the (sexed) body is discursively and linguistically constructed,[2] where the body is inaccessible except through language. This does not mean that the material body does not exist,

> [f]or surely bodies live and die; eat and sleep; feel pain, pleasure; endure illness and violence; and these 'facts', one might skeptically proclaim, cannot be dismissed as mere construction. Surely there must be some kind of necessity that accompanies these primary and irrefutable experiences. And surely there is.
>
> (Butler 1993: xi).

Butler is not suggesting that the body is reducible to language, but rather, that (knowledge of) the body is only accessible through language. Butler (1993) argues that bodies are discursively constructed through materialisation and signification. The body comes to be known, to itself and others, through the materialisation of language, and that materialisation requires the reiterative process of (re)signification for the body to be perceived as a fact, as reality. Butler argues that the body represents '*a process of materialization that stabilizes over time to produce the effect of boundary, fixity and surface we call matter*' (1993: 9, italics in original). Butler (1993: 68) goes on to suggest that 'language and materiality are not opposed, for language both is and refers to that which is material, and what is material never fully escapes the process by which it is signified'. The body is not some linguistic effect; rather, as with gender, the body congeals into the semblance of an ontological reality through language/discourse. The sexed, gendered, and dis/abled body is therefore performative.

Performativity figures throughout this book. Performativity refers to the practices by which identities are produced and enacted through repeated acts. In the context of gender, it is

> the repeated stylization of the body, a set of repeated acts within a highly rigid regulatory frame that congeal over time to produce the appearance of substance, of a natural sort of being. A political genealogy of gender ontologies, if it is successful, will deconstruct the substantive appearance of gender into its constitutive acts and locate and account for those acts within the compulsory frames set by the various forces that police the social appearance of gender.
>
> (Butler 1990: 33)

Butler (1990) argues that gender is a verb rather than a noun, and that constructs assume an ontological reality through 'doing' social practice. I suggest that dis/ability is likewise performative, and more importantly, performativity can be enacted and produced to either consolidate or destabilise norms. The notion of performativity is useful in this book as I use it to illuminate the spaces where disabled people either consolidate or resist the (discursive) practices through which disabled embodiment is constituted.

While it is perhaps easy to see how gender is discursively constructed, the construction of disability may appear to be a little less obvious and a little more complicated. Indeed, many have critiqued the argument that disability, or impairment more specifically, is discursively constructed (see Shakespeare 2006, 2013; Shakespeare and Watson 1997; Siebers 2008; Vehmas and Mäkelä 2008). Shakespeare (2013: 73) embraces a critical realist perspective of disability and argues that 'impairment has always existed and has its own experiential reality'. While Shakespeare (2013) posits that post-structural disability theorists are more concerned with discourse than the material reality of disabled people's lives, I argue that this claim rests on a narrow definition of discourse. Discourse refers to more than language; discourse refers to 'practices that systematically form the objects of which they speak' (Foucault 1972: 54). Discourse, then, incorporates language and social practice, and refers to the meanings, statements, and representations that congeal to create a particular version of 'reality'. Edwards, Ashmore, and Potter (1995: 26) note that these relativist/realist debates typically devolve into realists who thump on furniture and mention death and the existence of rocks, seeking to highlight a 'reality that *cannot* be denied' (italics in original). Yet Edwards, Ashmore, and Potter (1995: 27) suggest that

> [a]ll the pointings to, demonstrations of and descriptions of brute reality are inevitably semiotically mediated and communicated ... The very act of producing a non-represented, unconstructed external world is inevitably representational ...

Drawing upon the metaphorical example of those who thump furniture or talk about the existence of rocks, Edwards, Ashmore, and Potter (1995: 30) continue their argument by claiming that

> rocks are cultural too, in that they are categorized, included in the definition of the natural world, classified into sedimentary and igneous, divided into grains of sand, pieces of gravel, pebbles, stones, rocks, boulders, mountains, domesticated in parks and ornamental gardens, protected in wilderness, cut, bought, used and displayed as 'precious stones', and include as a subcategory 'girls' best friend'; not to mention coolant for vodka!

Edwards, Ashmore, and Potter (1995) do not deny the materiality of rocks, they merely seek to highlight that the meaning of that materiality is constructed through various technologies/discourses/practices and in different temporalities and spatialities.

To be clear, I do not deny the materiality of the body. Rather, I am arguing that the material body is made intelligible/recognisable as a particular sort of body through discursive practices. Just as Butler (1990) argued that sex was always already gender, I suggest the division between 'biological' impairment and 'social' disability ignores that the social disabled body and the impaired body are both materialised through social (re)signification. Following Butler (1993) and Tremain (2002: 42; 2015), I argue that impairment is discursively constructed, and that 'impairment has been disability all along'. My intention in this book, then, is to shift the emphasis from the individual body to the social practices through which disabled people are constituted. If we accept that impairment is a *disabled* category (in the same way that sex is naturalised as a *gendered* category)—which critical realists accept (Shakespeare and Watson 1997; Siebers 2008)—then there can be no (onto)logical distinction between impairment and disability (Corker 1999; Tremain 2002).

The edifice upon which the impairment/disability distinction is built is fundamentally unstable (Butler 1990), and the establishment (and maintenance) of these categories works to maintain compulsory abledness in an ableist culture (McRuer 2002, 2006). Tremain (2015: 14) suggests that over the past two centuries, a vast apparatus has been established to secure what is understood as normal in the general population, and this has caused

> the contemporary disabled subject to emerge into discourse and social existence ... These (and a host of other) practices, procedures, and policies have created, classified, codified, managed, and controlled social anomalies through which some people have been divided from others and objectivised as (for instance) physically impaired, insane, handicapped, mentally ill, retarded, or deaf.

The practices of division and classification 'from others produce the illusion of impairment [and disability]' (Tremain 2002: 42). If impairment and disability are cultural constructions that define and shape the body, how is the disabled body/subject materialised in the flesh?

The disabled subject

In order to consider how a body becomes 'disabled', I turn to Butler's (1993) notion of subjectivation. Theorising subjectivity opens up possibilities for thinking about bodies otherwise, and to consider the disciplinary and discursive practices through which the disabled subject comes into being. I specifically draw upon Butler's (1993) work with Althusser's concept of interpellation, which refers to how subjectivities are conferred, and then assumed or embodied, through action. Butler (1993) cites Althusser's example of a police officer hailing an individual in the street, proclaiming 'Hey, you there!' (Althusser 1971: 174). When the individual turns to acknowledge the hail, they become a subject (or subjectivated) as the individual has recognised that it was them being hailed (Althusser 1971: 174). Importantly for Butler, this subjectivation can happen even when the person hailed refuses to turn, or does not hear the hail. Butler (1993: 7–8) applies Althusser's account of interpellation to the construction of sex and gender:

> [c]onsider the medical interpellation which (the recent emergence of the sonogram notwithstanding) shifts an infant from an 'it' to a 'she' or a 'he,' and in that naming, the girl is 'girled,' brought into the domain of language and kinship through the interpellation of gender. But that 'girling' of the girl does not end there; on the contrary, that founding interpellation is reiterated by various authorities and throughout various intervals of time to reenforce or contest this naturalized effect. The naming is at once the setting of a boundary, and also the repeated inculcation of a norm.

As Butler argues, the naming of a girl is an interpellative, performative act that designates a sex and gender to a body that becomes intelligible through discourse. To remain a viable subject, through adherence to normative regimes of intelligibility, the body must be brought into the world and 'girled' (Butler 1993). The naming of the girl is not a statement of fact; it is cultural imposition that is perceived to be natural. What is considered 'natural' will 'not only produce the domain of intelligible bodies, but produce as well a domain of unthinkable, abject, unlivable bodies' (Butler 1993: xi).

Impairment/disability, I argue, operates in the same way as the 'girling' above. Notwithstanding the fact that any subject can be interpellated as disabled at any point (meaning that anyone can become disabled), the act of naming the impaired/disabled body is a medical interpellative, performative statement that constitutes the (disabled) body in a particular way:

[a]t the moment of interpellation, the very act of 'naming' the impairment immediately triggers an entire semiotic chain of meaning that draws on an already historically situated discourse that links 'impairment' with the 'defective body' that needs to be 'normalized' rather than a 'different body' that has 'different' needs.

(Erevelles 2016: 24)

For example, when a person is interpellated as disabled, they immediately enter a repertoire of discourses that mark disabled bodies as outside the norm, and they are subjected, and in many cases segregated, according to that performative act. The discursive construction of disability then leads to material acts and consequences that are embodied and performed by the subject interpellated as disabled. It would be a mistake, however, to presume that the act of interpellation is deterministic. While we cannot necessarily choose the terms within which we become interpellated, discourse provides for 'something we might call agency, the repetition of an originary subordination for another purpose, one whose future is partially open' (Butler 1997: 38).

The fact that interpellation is a performative act, too, implies that the terms under interrogation are reiterable, and potentially contestable and changeable (Butler 1993). These points are important, because as I position disabled people in relation to the abject, I am also interested in opening up spaces of possibility where abjection can be resisted/reclaimed, and the terms of intelligibility reimagined. This is a politics that moves away from a medical account of disability and a victim/perpetrator paradigm of violence towards a theorisation of disability as social, contingent, and revisable; it is a politics framed through a theorisation of disability as abjection.

The abject

In the previous sections I have addressed the body and its materiality in order to illustrate that disability is discursively constructed, and that this construction is positioned outside the norm of the healthy/abled body. One question this raises both in the context of this book's project and more generally is: *What is the relationship between the materiality of the body and the matter of bodies in political terms?* In a similar vein, Butler (1993: 16) asks,

[h]ow does the materialization of the norm in bodily formation produce a domain of abjected bodies, a field of deformation, which, in failing to qualify as the fully human, fortifies those regulatory norms? What challenge does that excluded and abjected realm produce to a symbolic hegemony that might force a radical rearticulation of what qualifies as bodies that matter, ways of living that count as 'life,' lives worth protecting, lives worth saving, lives worth grieving?

The discursive construction of bodies renders some bodies intelligible and others unintelligible. The terms of this intelligibility are figured through norms that constitute bodies as more or less normal, more or less human. Warner (1999: 53) notes,

> [n]early everyone, it seems, wants to be normal. And who can blame them, if the alternative is being abnormal, or deviant, or not being one of the rest of us? Put in those terms, there doesn't seem to be a choice at all.

As ability is naturalised/normalised throughout society, disability has become 'other', or abnormal and abject. Whether it be Siebers (2008) notion of the 'ideology of ability', McRuer's (2002, 2006) 'compulsory able-bodiedness', or a resignification of Butler's (1990) *Gender Trouble* as *Ability Trouble*, disability has been positioned as unintelligible and outside the norm(al). I am interested in this constitution of a space or zone outside the norm, and to theorise abjection as a social practice and embodied experience that positions the disabled body outside the norm *and at the same time* opens up possibilities for dissolution of the boundaries through which this outside is materialised.

In the discussion that follows, I give an account of the theory of the abject as the central frame in this book, and apply it to an examination of the processes and experiences of violence against disabled people. Young (1990: 142) suggests that a theory of the abject 'offers a means of understanding behavior and interactions that express group-based fear or loathing'. Tyler (2013: 3, 4) also argues that 'there has been no sustained account of abjection as a lived social process', and that within existing accounts, there is an omission 'of what it means to be (made) abject, to be one who repeatedly finds herself the object of the other's objectifying disgust'. My aim is to address this lacuna, and to explore the social and psychic instances in which disabled people experience abjection, and abjectify themselves.

Specifically, I develop an account of abjection to explore the ways in which disabled bodies are rendered unintelligible, and are violated through various technologies/practices. The abject has multiple forms and dimensions and is a difficult and slippery concept to describe and define (Tyler 2013; Warin 2010). There is also a conflation between the terms 'abject' and 'abjection', and a lack of understanding that they represent different processes and states. For example, the abject refers to a subject position, yet abjection refers to an act or process. Yet, as a concept, abjection 'allows us to think about forms of violence and social exclusion on multiple scales and from multiple dimensions' (Tyler 2013: 21). As my theoretical interest in abjection emerged in the early stages of this project, I turned to Kristeva's (1982) *Powers of Horror: An Essay on Abjection*, as it offers perhaps the most sustained account of the abject (Creed 1993; Cregan 2006; Rudge 2015; Tyler 2013).

Abjection, for Kristeva (1982), is a crisis of the self where one violently casts off or expunges that which threatens subjective integrity/identity. Abjection is a psychic and bodily reaction to threats to the subject's borders, and functions to preserve the subject (Kristeva 1982). The abject is a source of horror; it is neither subject nor object, and it is simultaneously repulsive and fascinating (Kristeva 1982). Kristeva (1982: 2) cites multiple examples that precipitate 'a discharge, a convulsion, a crying out', such as a corpse, blood, vomit, shit, menses, and so on. I add to this list: disability.

While Kristeva never mentions disability in her text (1982), I extend her account to incorporate disability. After all, disabled people are abjected by abled people as frightening, tragic, pitiable, or unlucky (Dohmen 2016; Hughes 2009). In this way, disability itself becomes the source of abjection for many disabled people, and this is because disability is not only constituted as repulsive and disgusting, but also as a biological abnormality that befalls people. Many disabled people internalise these beliefs:

> [f]rom the moment a child is born, he/she emerges into a world where he/she receives messages that to be disabled is to be *less than*, a world where disability may be *tolerated* but in the *final instance*, is *inherently negative*.
> (Campbell 2009a: 17, italics in original)

Such negative attitudes about disability are partly induced, I argue, by ableism. I am guided by Campbell's (2017: 287–288, italics in original) definition of ableism as a

> system of causal relations about the order of life that produces processes and systems of entitlement and exclusion. This causality fosters conditions of microaggression, internalized ableism and, in their jostling, notions of (un)encumbrance. A system of dividing practices, ableism institutes the reification and classification of populations. Ableist systems involve the *differentiation*, *ranking*, *negation*, *notification* and *prioritization* of sentient life.

Ableism is based on the premise that the abled body is natural and normal, 'the corporeal standard', 'species-typical and therefore essential and fully human' body (Campbell 2001: 44). Ableist assumptions, practices, and beliefs reign supreme, producing *disablism* (the belief that disabled people constitute inferior ways of being), and works to constitute disabled bodies as abject. As Campbell (2008) cautions us, ableism and disablism should not be used interchangeably or conflated, for they 'render quite radically different understandings of the status of disability to the norm' (2009a: 5). Ableism produces ideals surrounding abledness, while disablism produces ideals surrounding disability (Campbell 2009b). Given that both disabled and abled people are shaped by ableism, disabled subjectivity is constituted as an abject state.

Throughout the progress of the research contained in this book, I continually reflected upon Kristeva's account of the abject. While it is useful to the extent that I have just described, I ultimately became frustrated with it for two reasons. First, because of Kristeva's ahistorical, universalist, and psychoanalytic account, there is an omission of the social dimension of abjection. Specifically, Kristeva's (1982) conception does not account for the abjection of bodies in (symbolic/physical) social terms; only in bodily and psychic terms. Second, I became concerned with what I saw as the limits of her account, especially in relation to possibilities for both individual and collective resistance. I found myself preoccupied with such questions as: *If certain populations are abject, are they forever abject? Are there sites of resistance?* Commingling with this period, I engaged with Butler's work on abjection (1990, 1993, in Meijer and Prins 1998), and found it useful in extending my theorisation of abjection and grounding it in a more sociological and political account. Despite the problems with her work, I incorporate Kristeva's psychic account of abjection with Butler's more social, philosophical, and political account (described more fully in Chapter 2). In this way, I explore abjection as a simultaneously psychic and social process.

Fortuitously, during the later stages of the project, I stumbled upon McClintock's (1995) work on abjection. McClintock (1995: 72) suggests there are seven dimensions of abjection: abject *objects*, abject *states*, abject *zones*, *agents* of abjection, socially abjected *groups*, *psychic* processes of abjection, and *political* processes of abjection. McClintock's (1995) work helped me conjoin Kristeva and Butler's account of abjection, and in this book I use McClintock's framework, informed by Kristeva, Butler and others, to account for the multiple dimensions abjection takes, and the ways in which various practices/technologies regulate the (disabled) subject. I also consider how abjection is produced and reproduced, socially and psychically. This approach to theorising abjection became critical as I reflected on the stories of the research participants.

In November 2015, I interviewed one participant, *Warren Goodwin*, a second time, and in reflecting on this encounter I was struck by how McClintock's (1995) multi-dimensional account of abjection could inform my analysis. Warren and I met at a self-advocacy group for disabled people —an abject *zone*. Prior to the interview, he asked me to get a sandwich out of his bag. In addition to the label intellectual disability, Warren also has cerebral palsy. He spends most of life in a wheelchair (an abject *object*), and according to ableist norms, has poor mobility, slurred speech, and dribbles. I retrieved the chicken and lettuce sandwich from his bag, unwrapped it, and placed it next to his hands. As Warren picked it up and started to eat it, chicken and lettuce fell from the sandwich, as well as from his mouth. He chewed with his mouth wide open, and I watched as he masticated the food. Food dribbled down his chin. In these moments, the sandwich, for me, transformed into an abject *object*. I found it repulsive, and I gagged; twice. My gag was a *psychic process* of abjection; it was unconscious and unintentional, and I became an *agent* of abjection by abjectifying Warren to preserve my own bodily integrity. If Warren had noticed my response—and

I am not sure that he did—he may have felt abjected, rejected, disgusting. I felt a profound sense of shame with this encounter, and I laboured over the event and the feelings it evoked for weeks without telling anybody. My shame was an abject *state*.

In using McClintock's (1995) approach to abjection to reflect on this encounter, I not only saw the multiple dimensions abject/ion takes, but also understood how abjection is shared and relational. Throughout this book, I build upon this relational account of abjection in order to expose the various discourses, practices, and technologies through which we might understand the ways in which disabled bodies are abjected by abled people. This relational account of abjection is critical to the theorisation that informs this book and my reflections on the life history narratives of the thirteen people who participated in the interviews.

The life history method

The term 'life history' is deployed rather loosely in this book, and for a considerable period of time I was referring to them as 'life stories'. There is considerable disagreement in the literature about the terms (Denzin 1989); some scholars use life story and life history interchangeably (Atkinson 1998; Plummer 2004), while others place different emphasis upon each (Denzin 1989). For example, Atkinson (1998: 8) says there is 'little difference' between the two terms, and that they are 'usually different terms for the same thing'. In contrast, however, Goodson and Sikes (2001) suggest that life stories come under the umbrella of life histories, where the former looks at life experiences, but the latter situates these experiences within broader social contexts. Roberts (2002) adds another qualification, suggesting that the life story is narrated from the viewpoint of the participant, whereas the life history is presented and interpreted by the researcher. I chose not to confine myself to any strict method or interpretation throughout the research process, but rather chose to borrow and conjoin various elements from different approaches I thought were most suited to my own research. In the following section I introduce some concepts about the nature of the life history method that helped guide my project.

Atkinson (1998: 8) suggests that a life history/story is a

> story a person chooses to tell about the life he or she has lived, told as completely and honestly as possible, what is remembered of it, and what the teller wants others to know of it, usually as a result of a guided interview by another.

This proved a useful working definition in the earlier stages of my research. Plummer (2001) suggests there are two types of life histories: short and long. For Plummer (2001), a long life history would be gathered over many interviews and a significant passage of time, and can be complemented by interviews with other people or the analysis of other documents. As I reflected on the reality and time constraints of my doctoral research, coupled with the idea that I was interviewing people who had traumatic stories to share, I did not want to needlessly prolong their participation. Contrasting the long life history, Plummer (2001) suggests short life histories can be completed within the space of thirty minutes to three hours. Given the communication barriers I anticipated between myself and the participants, I decided to interview each participant up to four times, with each interview lasting about an hour. I stress here that much disability research, either implicitly or explicitly, places communication barriers squarely upon people labelled 'intellectually disabled'. Taking a different approach, I argue that it is my own weaknesses in communicating differently, as well as an ableist and disablist society that invisibilises disabled people from public spaces—and therefore minimising engagement and communication between disabled and abled people—that propagates these differences as problems.

Plummer (2001) makes a further distinction among different types of life histories, suggesting there are naturalistic, researched, and reflexive interviews. *Naturalistic* life histories involve stories that people tell in a natural and unmediated way, and Plummer (2001) provides the autobiography as an example. In contrast, *researched* life histories refer to stories that are collected for research purposes, where broader social themes and issues are compared and analysed (Plummer 2001). Last, and building upon the researched life history method, *reflexive* life histories add a greater degree of awareness about the discursive construction of a life history (Plummer 2001). Plummer (2001: 34) suggests that reflexive life histories 'do not simply tell the tale of a life', but rather illustrate the 'messiness', as Law (2004) might call it, and constructed nature of meaning, experience, and subjectivity. The researched and reflexive approaches to life histories informed this research.

Another point of clarification for Plummer (2001) is the distinction between the life history as a resource and a topic. In the former approach, the life history is seen as a resource that constructs an understanding of social life and phenomena. For example, Dowsett's (1996) account of gay men's sexuality and sexual practices during the AIDS crisis in Australia involved the life histories of twenty gay men. In contrast, the life history as a topic takes life histories as a subject of inquiry, asking such questions as why people tell their stories, how they tell their stories, and how spatial and temporal factors affect the different versions of the stories they tell. These are methodological and epistemological questions, and I see no reason why 'resource' and 'topic' life histories are mutually exclusive.[3] Indeed, my aim in this research is to privilege the experiential accounts of the research participants, whilst also exposing the various methodological considerations inherent to life history work. Given that many of the participants in this research had already participated in research, or had told their stories in adversarial or prosecutorial encounters, it was also interesting to see how many of the participants shaped their stories as a resource and a topic.

Against this backdrop, Atkinson (1998) suggests some possible themes and topics to explore in a life history. He also stresses that questions need to be open-ended rather than closed so that answers are developed and detailed (Atkinson 1998). Atkinson (1998: 41, italics in original) also argues that the '*less structure a life story interview has, the more effective it will be* in achieving the goal of getting the person's own story in the way, form, and style that the individual wants to tell it in'. This epistemological, ethical, and political position privileges the participants' approach to the research interviews. Atkinson (1998) provides a suggested framework, comprising one hundred and thirty-four questions and seventy-nine sub-questions within eleven thematic clusters, but he stresses this is not exhaustive and is only intended as a general guide (see his text for the full list). The themes he selected include:

- birth and family of origin
- cultural setting and traditions
- social factors
- education
- love and work
- historical events and periods
- retirement
- inner life and spiritual awareness
- major life themes
- vision of the future
- closure questions (Atkinson 1998).

I found these categories and questions entirely normative and in some respects unhelpful for a non-normative research population. The list of questions was subsequently revised and adapted (with new questions added) to better reflect the research population.[4] I also rephrased many questions to ensure they were accessible for the participant, and this involved shortening questions for clarity, changing complex words to make them more accessible, avoiding or removing jargon, and keeping questions short yet simultaneously open-ended. Importantly, not all of the questions were asked, and I did not perceive these questions to be a 'checklist' that I must get through. Rather, in each interview some of the questions acted as prompts when required.

The interview approach I adopted was semi-structured and largely flexible. Yet this changed throughout the progress of the project. The early interviews were much more structured, which I attribute to my own nervousness. As fieldwork progressed, however, I became more confident and relaxed about the interview process, such that I was happy to explore any avenue of conversation the participants' initiated.

The participants

To assist the reader in clearly differentiating between the thirteen people who participated in this project, I provide brief biographies below, arranged in the order in which I met them. Pseudonyms are used for all participants:[5]

Lisa Austin is a 34-year-old woman, and she lives in Melbourne. She has a 6-year-old daughter, Stephanie, and is separated from the child's father. She has a history of child abuse from her mother, was bullied at school, and experienced people saying to her that she should not have had a child. Lisa promotes self-advocacy for people labelled 'intellectually disabled'.

Roger Cobb is a 67-year-old man who lives in Melbourne. Born in England before moving to Melbourne as a small child, Roger has spent most of his life in and out of asylums.[6] He has experienced violence and abuse at multiple points in his life. Today he spends his time involved in the self-advocacy movement.

Deb is a 54-year-old woman who was born in Melbourne. She spent almost all her youth in asylums, and has a traumatic history of sexual and physical violence. Deb discovered she is Indigenous[7] in 2009, and she has reconnected with her family. Deb goes to several disability organisations when she wants to socialise; otherwise, she is happy living her life on her own.

Jake Hawkins is a 22-year-old man who was born and lives in Sydney, and most of what he told me revolved around school bullying. Today he is involved in a transition programme in the hope that he might soon get a reliable job. He lives with his parents and has a girlfriend. After our first interview, Jake did not want to participate further.

Anne-Marie Holloway is a 43-year-old woman who resides in Sydney. Throughout our interviews Anne-Marie mostly focussed on a series of incidents with the police, who discriminated against her when she reported domestic violence. Now that these two events are behind her, Anne-Marie enjoys going to the beach, spending time with her dad, horse riding, sewing, and catching up with friends for coffee.

Amal Alam is a 35-year-old Lebanese-Australian woman who lives in Sydney with her family. In addition to the label 'intellectual disability', Amal is blind. She experienced a significant amount of bullying during her schooling, and she still experiences daily harassment from strangers. Amal works at both a sheltered workshop and does administration at another business, and this keeps her busy; otherwise, she enjoys socialising with her friends and travelling.

Emma Silva is a 32-year-old woman who was born in England, and moved to Sydney with her mum when she was 6 months old. Now living with her aunt and uncle, Emma is currently looking for employment, which she struggles to find due to discrimination. To develop her skills, Emma regularly goes to TAFE (Technical and Further Education), and in her free time she goes to the movies with her friends, or catches up with them for coffee.

Freddie Watkins is a 50-year-old man who lives in Sydney. He has a son, who is 8 years old, but his ex-wife will not let Freddie see him. Freddie lives alone, and his neighbours do not socialise with him. Freddie says he prefers this because he likes to be alone. He has been bashed once, and his house has been robbed. After one interview, Freddie drew his participation in this research to a close.

Joshua Rodgers is a 24-year-old man and he lives between his mum and dad's houses in Sydney. He is involved in self-advocacy, and he goes to TAFE. Joshua focussed a lot of his story on his experiences at school, where the other students bullied him. Joshua also identifies as bisexual, and this has caused some apprehension for him in the past. Joshua has had his learner driver's license for three years now, and he will soon go for his provisional license once he has more time to practice.

Peter Camilleri is a 57-year-old man who has spent his entire life living in Sydney. He experienced bullying at school, and he has also been bullied by his friends and family. Peter is a truck driver, and he has been in a relationship with his partner for 15 years. He likes going to the speedway with her to watch car racing, and going to the local club to have dinner, a drink, and play on the pokies (poker machines).

Warren Goodwin is 58 years old and he lives in Melbourne. When we met, Warren only wanted to talk about two things: being gay and the sexual assault he experienced. After two interviews, Warren ended his participation in this research.

Richard Brady is a 60-year-old man, and father of three children. He lives in Sydney, and is now divorced from his children's mother. Richard grew up in an asylum, but these days he does not like talking about it. Richard has been bashed and bullied throughout his life, and today he is involved in self-advocacy work.

Clifton Murphy is a 55-year-old man who lives in Sydney. One of two children, Clifton was severely neglected by his parents growing up. In light of this neglect, Clifton surrounds his life with animals. He has worked as an animal technician and had jobs at pounds, zoos, and wildlife and national parks. He has been married and divorced, and Clifton considers his life a daily struggle.

These thirteen people contributed parts of their lives to this book, and for that I am forever grateful. Their stories appear throughout the body of this book, sometimes briefly, sometimes completely, as the tropes and theories within this work unfold. Their stories are deployed to illuminate the theoretical constructs central to this research and its ambition of reimagining disablist and ableist violence as abjection, and finding scales of resistance.

The one in the many, and the many in the one

Drawing from Bansel (2012) and Butler (2005), it is my imperative to resist the power of number as a standard-bearer for reliability, validity, and significance in research. In this book, I work with the thirteen life histories I have collected in order to build my account of abjection. I argue that any one of these accounts is made possible through multiple constitutive relations, and is, as such, an assemblage of many accounts, such that each account is simultaneously collective and singular (Bansel 2012). In this way, I do not merely consider one account to be an example, or representative, of many, but rather, consider one account to represent one *and* many simultaneously. Butler (2005: 7, 8) writes that

> there is no 'I' that can fully stand apart from the social conditions of its emergence, no 'I' that is not implicated in a set of conditioning moral norms, which, being norms, have a social character that exceeds a purely personal or idiosyncratic meaning ... the 'I' has no story of its own that is not also the story of a relation—or set of relations—to a set of norms.

Each of the participants have lives that are particular to them, and while they have experienced highly individualised events, 'any single account of experience is always an account of other times, places, subjects and practices' (Bansel 2012: 7). In the accounts I give of the narratives of the people who participated in this project, I emphasise the relational and simultaneous constitution of the individual and social body.

Given this approach to the thirteen life history narratives as simultaneously individual and collective, psychic and social, I interrogate what abjection, as a lived social process, looks like. I expose the ways in which the disabled subjects experience(d) abjection, and abjected themselves (and others). Importantly, however, my aim is to animate these lived experiences of abjection in order to speculate upon how abjection might be resisted. I argue that without exploring how abjection is lived as a social process, it is impossible to explore the spaces of possibility within which abjection might be resisted, and the terms of intelligibility reimagined. To position disabled people in relation to the abject is not enough; exposing experiences of abjection, thinking otherwise about disability, and opening up spaces of possibility in which abjection can be resisted or reclaimed are all critical to reimagining disablist and ableist violence as abjection.

My position in the research

The title of the subheading above, along with the ways in which the preceding parts of this book have been written, signals my approach and understanding of the ways in which I position myself in relation to this project. Most objectivist/positivist research privileges the objective production of knowledge to resolve a problem with an identified 'fact', which is identified through techniques such as the experimental method—and reliance upon dependent and independent variables, reliability, and validity. In keeping with my post-structural position, I contest these claims to objectivity and validity (Foucault 1970). In efforts to portray strictly objectivist knowledge, many scholars avoid first-person language—as if the research itself, and discussion of it, magically appeared on the page without the participation of a human agent. Haraway (1991: 189) calls this the 'god trick': the 'seeing everything from nowhere', of making the author disappear, of presenting the text as 'unbiased' and 'objective'. Instead, I recognise my complicity in the creation of knowledge and conduct of research. As Denzin (1989: 61) writes, the researcher's 'own experiences provide the most important source of data for their theories'. I recognise my own background, subjectivity, positionality, and biases have influenced this project, and as Reinharz (1992) invites, I acknowledge and reflect upon these factors.

Specifically, as a gay man, I often perceive and locate disability issues through the prism of heterosexism. This has its benefits and its drawbacks. To begin with, I know what abjection, oppression, and violence looks and feels like. Yet this is funnelled through the lens of gender and sexuality, not dis/ability. I have never individually experienced disability, and throughout this project I often had moments where I was confronted by my own able-ism. Yet, in some ways, we have all experienced disability. As Titchkosky (2003) acknowledges, while she has dyslexia, she also experiences blindness because she shares a life with Rod Michalko, who is blind. Titchkosky (2003) is aware of the experiences that blind and dyslexic people go through. Growing up with a disabled sister, I am acutely aware of the experiences she and I have observed and felt in negotiating an ableist society. Importantly, disability experience is relational, and everyone shapes the meaning of 'disabled identity' (Titchkosky 2003).

At a broader level, too, I recognise my own privilege and abled position in this research. In positioning myself in this research, I identify as *temporarily abled*. This acknowledges the slipperiness of dis/ability, and the realisation that disability may enter my own embodied/corporeal life. I realise that this term is problematic, however, as I may never become interpellated as disabled. Nevertheless, I choose to foreground the possibility in order to destabilise any perception that abledness is a fixed and final position.

Speaking about them—not *for* them, and not *as* them

Earlier I suggested that some life histories told from the viewpoint of the participant are collaborative (Roberts 2002). That is, the participant and researcher collaborate to produce the life history in its written form (Goodley 2000). Plummer (2001: 177) encourages the researcher to

> get your subject's own words, really come to grasp them from the inside, and then yourself turn it into a structured and coherent statement that uses the subject's words in places and the social scientist's in others but does not lose their authentic meaning.

Given that I find this quest for authenticity problematic, I approached it in a different way. Rather than speak *as* the participants or *for* them, I chose to speak *about* them. Alcoff (1991: 7) argues that the practice of 'speaking for or on behalf of less privileged persons has actually resulted (in many cases) in increasing or reinforcing the oppression of the group spoken for'. While I am a gay man—and consequently oppressed because of my non-normative sexuality—my gender, middle-class status, Anglo background, and (temporary) abledness position me in the liminal status of insider-outsider, or what Heilman (1980) coins, 'native-as-stranger'. While I may understand the experiences of oppression based upon identity, I nevertheless argue that speaking for others is a problematic, and potentially unethical, practice (Alcoff 1991). I reject the idea that I could ever speak *for* anyone or *as* anyone, so throughout this book I have provided unaltered narrative excerpts from the participants who are too often denied the status of subjects. Given that one of my aims was to foreground the participants' experiences of violence, I worked to render their experiences visible in order to make such experiences available to interpretation and theorisation. Ultimately, the participants were asked to speak *as* disabled people, and speaking *about* them enables me to avoid the idea that I could ever possibly speak *for* them.

Yet I also recognise that in de- and re-contextualising their narratives, and opening up spaces for theorisation, I may also be enacting a form of symbolic violence. Alcoff (1991: 9, italics in original) suggests that

> [i]n both the practice of speaking for as well as the practice of speaking about others, I am engaging in the act of representing the other's needs, goals, situation, and in fact, *who they are*. I am representing them *as* such and such, or in post-structuralist terms, I am participating in the construction of their subject-positions. The act of representation cannot be understood as founded on an act of discovery wherein I discover their true selves and then simply relate my discovery. I will take it as a given that such representations are in every case mediated and the product of interpretation.

Accepting this fact, I nevertheless cannot retreat from it. Alcoff (1991: 8) asks herself, 'if I don't speak for those less privileged than myself, am I abandoning my political responsibility to speak out against oppression, a responsibility incurred by the very fact of my privilege?' More fundamentally, Spivak (1990: 59) argues that 'the question "Who should speak?" is less crucial than "Who will listen?"'. Alcoff (1991: 29) also suggests that in interpreting and speaking for/about others, it is vital to ask, 'will it enable the empowerment of oppressed peoples?' My answer: I hope so.

Overview of the book

A story unfolds in the following chapters that, in addition to exploring abjection, seek to imagine disability otherwise. In Chapter 2, 'Social Abjection and Reappropriation', I introduce Butler's (1993, in Meijer and Prins 1998) notion of the abject and argue how it better accounts for the political and social dynamics of abjection as a lived social process. I also speculatively turn to the notion of reappropriation in the context of disability in an effort to think of ways in which abjection can be reimagined. In Chapter 3, 'Deb's Narrative:

Exploring the Multi-Dimensional Forms of Abjection', I introduce Deb and her life history narrative, and consider the abjection she has experienced throughout her life. In building an account of abjection, I specifically interrogate how various dimensions of abjection come together in particular temporal and spatial moments, and explore how abjection is distributed, cyclical, compounding, and often invisibly inflicted on disabled bodies. In Chapter 4, 'Roger's Narrative: Abjection Amidst Chaos and Fragmentation', I continue to build my account of abjection through an exploration of Roger and his life history. Counterpoised with Deb's life history narrative, I consider how similar and distinct forms of abjection result in dis/similar experiences and outcomes in certain temporal/spatial contexts.

Following these separate chapters devoted to Deb and Roger, Chapter 5 'Eleven Lives' provides biographical details of the other eleven people who participated in the research. I do this in order to introduce the reader to the remaining participants, and to contextualise Chapter 6. In Chapter 6, '(Psychic) Self-Abjection: Pathologisation and Disavowal', I examine the ways in which disabled subjects pathologise and disavow their own disabled subjectivities. Whereas Deb and Roger's chapters explore abjection in largely social terms, this chapter examines the interiorisation of the social into, and as, one's psychic life. In Chapter 7, 'Anne-Marie's Narrative: Abjection and Resistance', I work with Anne-Marie's narrative to consolidate my account of abjection as simultaneously social and psychic, individual and collective. Most importantly, however, I explore the conditions in which abjection can be resisted or reclaimed. Finally, in Chapter 8, 'Reflections, Possibilities, and Resistance', I bring together the multiple threads that constitute the argument of the book and consider several implications for abjection and abject bodies. I start by exploring several stories in which disabled people have resisted their abjection, and move to consider a coalitional, relational ethics where abjection might be resisted through collective practice. I argue that theorising abjection in this way has made it possible to identify the circumstances in which abjection might possibly be resisted and the terms of disability un/intelligibility reimagined.

Conclusion

In this chapter I have begun to map the origins and emergent directions of this book. I have introduced a preliminary understanding of the abject, and I build upon this throughout each of the remaining chapters. While I seek to privilege the accounts of the disabled people who participated in my project, I contextualise their experiences within broader discussions about prejudice, subjectivity, and normativity. The implications of this book are wide and varied; each participant's narrative speaks to the ways in which society views disabled people, how they view themselves, and how reductive approaches to different forms of embodiment can be viewed differently. In

Chapter 2, I consider these inquiries by interrogating the notion of the abject, and specifically examining the spaces of possibility in which abjection might be thought of differently.

Notes

1 In this book, I use the term abled to refer to (temporarily) non-disabled people. Yet, I simultaneously recognise that the term is created within normalising discourses and practices. I remain sceptical and questioning of the term, yet following Durie (2003), I also resist the temptation to use quotation marks to highlight the constructed and contested nature of this and other concepts. While this does require the reader to engage in the deconstruction of terms (I hope!), I cannot reconcile highlighting some words and not others at risk of suggesting some naturalness—and attendant normativity—around the unmarked terms.
2 This is an extension of her arguments from *Gender Trouble* (1990), where she argues that gender and sex are discursively constructed.
3 Plummer (2001) also acknowledges that these distinctions are not mutually exclusive.
4 This aligns with Atkinson's (1998) suggestion that the questions need to be considered in light of each particular person, and the research topic under investigation.
5 In referencing their age, I use the age they provided at the time of the interviews in 2015–2016.
6 While all of the participants in this research used the term '(disabled) institution', in this thesis I use the term 'asylum' to differentiate more clearly between different institutional spaces. Moreover, I use the term 'asylum' to be provocative, and to highlight that euphemistic changes in language do not address underlying social and cultural practices. 'Institution' is merely a new word that replaces the contaminated 'asylum', yet I argue that little has changed within social practice that actually differentiates between asylums and institutions (see Sinason 1992).
7 I use Deb's preferred terminology.

References

Alcoff, L 1991, 'The Problem of Speaking for Others', *Cultural Critique*, (20): 5–32.
Althusser, L 1971, 'Ideology and Ideological State Apparatuses (Notes Towards an Investigation)', in *Lenin and Philosophy and Other Essays*, edited by L Althusser, translated by B Brewster, Monthly Review Press, New York, pp. 127–186.
Atkinson, R 1998, *The Life Story Interview*, SAGE Publications, Thousand Oaks, CA.
Bansel, P 2012, 'Resisting and Re/counting the Power of Number: The One in the Many and the Many in the One', in *Discourse, Power, and Resistance down Under*, edited by M Vicars, T McKenna, and J White, Sense Publishers, Rotterdam, pp. 1–8.
Butler, J 1990, *Gender Trouble: Feminism and the Subversion of Identity*, Routledge, New York and London.
Butler, J 1993, *Bodies that Matter: On the Discursive Limits of 'Sex'*, Routledge, New York and London.
Butler, J 1997, *Excitable Speech: A Politics of the Performative*, Routledge, New York and London.
Butler, J 2004, *Precarious Life: The Powers of Mourning and Violence*, Verso, London and New York.
Butler, J 2005, *Giving an Account of Oneself*, Fordham University Press, New York.

Campbell, FAK 2001, 'Inciting Legal Fictions: "Disability's" Date with Ontology and the Ableist Body of the Law', *Griffith Law Review*, 10(1): 42–62.

Campbell, FAK 2008, 'Exploring Internalized Ableism Using Critical Race Theory', *Disability & Society*, 23(2): 151–162.

Campbell, FK 2009a, *Contours of Ableism: The Production of Disability and Abledness*, Palgrave Macmillan, London and New York.

Campbell, FK 2009b, 'Disability Harms: Exploring Internalized Ableism', in *Disabilities: Insights from across Fields and around the World, Volume 1, the Experience: Definitions, Causes, and Consequences*, edited by CA Marshall, E Kendall, ME Banks, and RMS Gover, Praeger Publishers, Westport, CT, pp. 19–33.

Campbell, FK 2012, 'Stalking Ableism: Using Disability to Expose "Abled" Narcissism', in *Disability and Social Theory: New Developments and Directions*, edited by D Goodley, B Hughes, and L Davis, Palgrave Macmillan, Basingstoke, Hampshire, UK, pp. 212–230.

Campbell, FK 2017, 'Queer Anti-sociality and Disability Unbecoming: An Ableist Relations Project?', in *New Intimacies, Old Desires: Law, Culture and Queer Politics in Neoliberal Times*, edited by O Sircar and D Jain, Zubaan, New Delhi, pp. 280–316.

Corker, M 1999, 'Differences, Conflations and Foundations: The Limits to "Accurate" Theoretical Representation of Disabled People's Experiences?', *Disability & Society*, 14(5): 627–642.

Creed, B 1993, *The Monstrous-Feminine: Film, Feminism, Psychoanalysis*, Routledge, London and New York.

Cregan, K 2006, *The Sociology of the Body: Mapping the Abstraction of Embodiment*, SAGE Publications, London.

Crenshaw, K 1991, 'Mapping the Margins: Intersectionality, Identity Politics, and Violence against Women of Colour', *Stanford Law Review*, 43(6): 1241–1299.

Denzin, NK 1989, *Interpretive Biography*, SAGE Publications, Newbury Park, CA.

Dohmen, J 2016, 'Disability as Abject: Kristeva, Disability, and Resistance', *Hypatia*, 31(4): 762–778.

Dowsett, GW 1996, *Practicing Desire: Homosexual Sex in the Era of AIDS*, Stanford University Press, Stanford, CA.

Durie, J 2003, 'Speaking the Silence of Whiteness', *Journal of Australian Studies*, 27 (79): 135–142.

Edwards, D, Ashmore, M, and Potter, J 1995, 'Death and Furniture: The Rhetoric, Politics and Theology of Bottom Line Arguments against Relativism', *History of the Human Sciences*, 8(2): 25–49.

Erevelles, N 2016, 'Deconstructing Difference: Doing Disability Studies in Multicultural Educational Contexts', in *Vital Questions Facing Disability Studies in Education*, 2nd, edition edited by S Danforth and SL Gabel, Peter Lang Publishing, New York, pp. 17–29.

Foucault, M 1970, *The Order of Things: An Archaeology of the Human Sciences*, Tavistock Publications, London.

Foucault, M 1972, *Archaeology of Knowledge*, translated by A.M Sheridan Smith, Routledge, London.

Fraser, N 2003, 'Social Justice in the Age of Identity Politics: Redistribution, Recognition, and Participation', in *Redistribution or Recognition? A Political—Philosophical Exchange*, edited by N Fraser and A Honneth, Verso, London and New York, pp. 7–109.

Galvin, R 2003, 'The Function of Language in the Creation and Liberation of Disabled Identities: From Saussure to Contemporary Strategies of Government', *Australian Journal of Communication*, 30(3): 83–100.

Goodley, D 2000, *Self-advocacy in the Lives of People with Learning Difficulties: The Politics of Resilience*, Open University Press, Buckingham and Philadelphia.

Goodley, D 2013, 'Dis/entangling Critical Disability Studies', *Disability & Society*, 28 (5): 631–644.

Goodley, D 2014, *Dis/ability Studies: Theorising Disablism and Ableism*, Routledge, London and New York.

Goodson, I and Sikes, P 2001, *Life History in Educational Settings: Learning from Lives*, Open University Press, Buckingham and Philadelphia.

Haraway, DJ 1991, *Simians, Cyborgs, and Women: The Reinvention of Nature*, Routledge, New York.

Heilman, SC 1980, 'Jewish Sociologist: Native-as-Stranger', *The American Sociologist*, 15(2): 100–108.

Hughes, B 2009, 'Wounded/Monstrous/Abject: A Critique of the Disabled Body in the Sociological Imaginary', *Disability & Society*, 24(4): 399–410.

Jacobs, JB and Potter, K 1998, *Hate Crimes: Criminal Law & Identity Politics*, Oxford University Press, New York.

Kristeva, J 1982, *Powers of Horror: An Essay on Abjection*, translated by LS Roudiez, Columbia University Press, New York.

Law, J 2004, *After Method: Mess in Social Science Research*, Routledge, New York.

Law, J and Singleton, V 2005, 'Object Lessons', *Organization*, 12(3): 331–355.

Mason-Bish, H 2013, 'Conceptual Issues in the Construction of Disability Hate Crime', in *Disability, Hate Crime and Violence*, edited by A Roulstone and H Mason-Bish, Routledge, London, pp. 11–24.

McClintock, A 1995, *Imperial Leather: Race, Gender and Sexuality in the Colonial Contest*, Routledge, New York and London.

McRuer, R 2002, 'Compulsory Able-Bodiedness and Queer/Disabled Existence', in *Disability Studies: Enabling the Humanities*, edited by SL Snyder, BJ Brueggemann, and R Garland Thomson, The Modern Language Association of America, New York, pp. 88–99.

McRuer, R 2006, *Crip Theory: Cultural Signs of Queerness and Disability*, New York University Press, New York and London.

Meekosha, H and Shuttleworth, R 2009, 'What's so "Critical" about Critical Disability Studies?', *Australian Journal of Human Rights*, 15(1): 47–76.

Meijer, IC and Prins, B (with J Butler) 1998, 'How Bodies Come to Matter: An Interview with Judith Butler', *Signs: Journal of Women in Culture and Society*, 23(2): 275–286.

Oliver, M 1996, *Understanding Disability: From Theory to Practice*, Macmillan, London.

Plummer, K 2001, *Documents of Life 2: An Invitation to Critical Humanism*, SAGE, London.

Plummer, K 2004, 'Life History Method', in *The SAGE Encyclopaedia of Social Science Research Methods, Volume 2*, edited by MS Lewis-Beck, A Bryman, and TF Liao, SAGE Publications, Thousand Oaks, CA, pp. 565–566.

Pratt, DP 1998, *Five Perspectives on Teaching in Adult and Higher Education*, Krieger Publishing, Malabar, FL.

Reinharz, S 1992, *Feminist Methods in Social Research*, Oxford University Press, New York.

Roberts, B 2002, *Biographical Research*, Open University Press, Buckingham and Philadelphia.

Rudge, T 2015, 'Julia Kristeva: Abjection, Embodiment and Boundaries', in *The Palgrave Handbook of Social Theory in Health, Illness and Medicine*, edited by F Collyer, Palgrave Macmillan, Basingstoke, Hampshire, pp. 504–519.

Shakespeare, T 2006, *Disability Rights and Wrongs*, Routledge, London and New York.

Shakespeare, T 2013, *Disability Rights and Wrongs Revisited*, 2nd, edition Routledge, London and New York.

Shakespeare, T and Watson, N 1997, 'Defending the Social Model', *Disability & Society*, 12(2): 293–300.

Shildrick, M 2009, *Dangerous Discourses of Disability, Subjectivity and Sexuality*, Palgrave Macmillan, Basingstoke, Hampshire.

Shildrick, M 2012, 'Critical Disability Studies: Rethinking the Conventions for the Age of Postmodernity', in *Routledge Handbook of Disability Studies*, edited by N Watson, A Roulstone, and C Thomas, Routledge, London and New York, pp. 30–41.

Siebers, T 2008, *Disability Theory*, The University of Michigan Press, Ann Arbor, MI.

Sinason, V 1992, *Mental Handicap and the Human Condition: An Analytic Approach to Intellectual Disability*, Free Association Books, London.

Slater, J 2015, *Youth and Disability: A Challenge to Mr Reasonable*, Ashgate Publishing, London.

Spivak, GC (with Sneja Gunew) 1990, 'Questions of Multi-Culturalism', in *The Post-Colonial Critic: Interviews, Strategies, Dialogues*, edited by S Harasym, Routledge, New York and London, pp. 59–66.

Titchkosky, T 2003, *Disability, Self, and Society*, University of Toronto Press, Toronto.

Tremain, S 2002, 'On the Subject of Impairment', in *Disability/Postmodernity: Embodying Disability Theory*, edited by M Corker and T Shakespeare, Continuum, London and New York, pp. 32–47.

Tremain, S 2015, 'Foucault, Governmentality, and Critical Disability Theory Today: A Genealogy of the Archive', in *Foucault and the Government of Disability*, 2nd, edition edited by S Tremain, The University of Michigan Press, Ann Arbor, pp. 9–23.

Tyler, I 2009, 'Against Abjection', *Feminist Theory*, 10(1): 77–98.

Tyler, I 2013, *Revolting Subjects: Social Abjection and Resistance in Neoliberal Britain*, Zed Books, London and New York.

Vehmas, S and Mäkelä, P 2008, 'A Realist Account of the Ontology of Impairment', *Journal of Medical Ethics*, 34(2): 93–95.

Warin, M 2010, *Abject Relations: Everyday Worlds of Anorexia*, Rutgers University Press, New Brunswick, NJ.

Warner, M 1999, *The Trouble with Normal: Sex, Politics, and the Ethics of Queer Life*, Harvard University Press, Cambridge, MA.

Young, IM 1990, *Justice and the Politics of Difference*, Princeton University Press, Princeton, NJ.

2 Social abjection and reappropriation

To reimagine disablist and ableist violence as abjection, the concepts under study must first be reconsidered. In the previous chapter, I outlined the development of my project and its movement from a construct of hate crime to the theory of the abject. Kristeva's (1982) theory of the abject was introduced as a starting point, and I also articulated some reservations about the extent to which it could inform the broader aims of the research contained within this book. While I appreciate Kristeva's account of abjection as a psychic and bodily process, I found its ahistorical and universalist dimensions—inherent to psychoanalysis—problematic both to my own theoretical position as a researcher and as a mode of framing the participants' narrated accounts in their experience. I did not, however, abandon the theory of the abject; to do so would have been pre-emptive. In fact, Kristeva's theory provided me the framework to develop an account of the abject more suited to my purposes, one informed by Butler (1990; 1993, in Meijer and Prins 1998). I am more sympathetic to Butler's theorisation not only because it provides a context for understanding the abjectification of disabled lives within socially and historically situated contexts, but also opens up spaces of possibility for resisting the imposition that disabled people are always and only abject.

In this chapter I introduce Butler's theory of the abject as it extends from the work in the previous chapter. I explain how Butler's account of the abject is useful in framing the everyday experiences of disabled people. More importantly, however, I go on to demonstrate how her theorisation opens up sites of resistance against abjection. Using critical disability studies and queer theory, I consider how disabled people might reappropriate the abjection they experience. My focus, then, is on how disabled people are rendered abject, yet possess the agency to resist these constructions.

Butler's theory of the abject

Butler first interrogates the notion of the abject in *Gender Trouble* (1990). The abject, according to Butler (1990: 133), designates that which has been expelled from the body, discharged as excrement, literally rendered 'Other'. This appears as an expulsion of alien elements, but the alien is effectively established through this expulsion. The construction of the 'not-me' as the abject establishes the boundaries of the body which are also the first contours of the subject.

Here Butler continues the Kristevan (1982) notion of the abject where it is seen as a psychic process, and (the borders of) the body are established through exclusion/expulsion. In her later work, Butler extends her theorisation of abjection beyond a psychoanalytic frame. Butler (1993) suggests that abjection is a discursive (rather than psychic) function that renders bodies unintelligible in political terms. Butler (1993: 3) writes that the

> exclusionary matrix by which subjects are formed thus requires the simultaneous production of a domain of abject beings, those who are not yet 'subjects', but who form the constitutive outside to the domain of the subject. The abject designates here precisely those 'unlivable' and 'uninhabitable' zones of social life which are nevertheless densely populated by those who do not enjoy the status of the subject, but whose living under the sign of the 'unlivable' is required to circumscribe the domain of the subject.

Butler (1993: 3) conceives that subjects are formed through exclusion/inclusion, and the abject emerges as the site 'against which—and by virtue of which—the domain of the subject will circumscribe its own claim to autonomy and to life'. For Butler (1993), then, the materialisation of an intelligible body/subject depends upon the simultaneous production of its antithesis: an unintelligible, abject body. Butler (1993: 3) continues:

> [i]n this sense, then, the subject is constituted through the force of exclusion and abjection, one which produces a constitutive outside to the subject, an abjected outside, which is, after all, 'inside' the subject as its own founding repudiation.

Butler (1993) argues that the process in which subjects establish their borders simultaneously functions as a mechanism to establish those bodies that matter and those that do not. The abject is a 'site of dreaded identification' that inhabits 'unlivable' and 'uninhabitable' zones of social life, while the subject inhabits liveable and inhabitable social zones (Butler 1993: 3). Importantly, the social production of a constitutive 'outside' simultaneously constitutes the 'inside' of the subject. In this way, there is a constitutive relation and movement between the external social body and the internal individual body; a movement between the social and the psychic.

Butler goes on to say that abject bodies are 'delegitimated bodies [that] fail to count as "bodies"', and that they are the 'constitutive outside' and 'nonnarrativizable' (1993: 15, 3, 188). As I understand it, Butler (1993) has *socialised* Kristeva's (1982) theory to consider the ways in which regulatory norms shape the political mattering and materialisation of bodies. According to Butler's (1993) discursive theorisation, the abject body can be considered a material construct of difference that is not discursively legitimate—it is literally all body and materiality without meaning. For Butler (1993), abjection refers to the process by which certain populations are excluded and rendered unintelligible as subjects because they fail to adhere to constructed normative ideals.

In a subsequent interview with Meijer and Prins (1998), Butler extends, clarifies, and socialises her theory of the abject again. Butler (in Meijer and Prins 1998: 277) writes,

> [t]he abjection of certain kinds of bodies, their inadmissibility to codes of intelligibility, does make itself known in policy and politics, and to live as such a body in the world is to live in the shadowy regions of ontology.

Abjection, then, for Butler becomes an ontological question where intelligible bodies count as real, and unintelligible bodies do not count at all; they are 'in some sense, unreal' (Lloyd 2007: 75). In the context of disability, abled bodies count as real within an ableist culture that constructs them as natural and intelligible, yet disabled bodies do not count because the ableist culture constructs them as *un*natural and *un*intelligible.

Butler's ontological suppositions about the abject as articulated above and in the context of her work more broadly have been queried by some scholars (see Lloyd 2008; Meijer and Prins 1998; White 1999). Lloyd (2008) suggests that there is a tension in Butler's work between her commitment to undermine ontological assumptions and her own ontological presuppositions. As documented above, Butler claims the abject lives in the 'shadowy regions of ontology' (in Meijer and Prins 1998: 277). To me, the question this raises is: *how can a body that fails to materialise still be a body?* Meijer and Prins (1998: 280) raise this tension with Butler, and suggest:

> [i]f you intend the concept of the 'abject' to refer to bodies that 'exist,' would it not be more adequate to say that, although abject bodies are constructed, have materialized, and gained intelligibility, they still fail to qualify as fully human? In other words, is it not the case that abject bodies do 'matter' ontologically and epistemologically but do not yet 'matter' in a normative-political sense?

Responding to this question, Butler (in Meijer and Prins 1998: 280) acknowledges that to say 'there are' abject bodies while simultaneously negating their claim to ontology is a 'performative contradiction'. Yet she goes on to suggest that she makes this contradiction on purpose, questioning how the 'domain of ontology is itself circumscribed by power' (1998: 280). For Butler, ontological effects are an instrument of power, and she is concerned with the ways in which these effects include and exclude, hierarchise and subordinate certain bodies.

Still, I question the terms of intelligibility Butler offers here, in particular how something unintelligible can nevertheless be intelligible even as it is only recognised as unintelligible. For something to be named unintelligible, must it not reach a level of intelligibility within discourse to accord it such recognition? While Kristeva (1982: 1) suggests the abject is 'neither subject nor object', would it not be more accurate to term the abject the unintelligible *subject?* Butler (in Meijer and Prins 1998: 281, italics in original) qualifies:

> it is not as if the unthinkable, the unintelligible has no discursive life; it *does* have one. It just lives within discourse as the radically uninterrogated and as the shadowy contentless figure for something that is not yet made real.

I appreciate this qualification because it illustrates the social contours of abjection (Schein 2000), where there is a 'differential production of the human or a differential materialization of the human' (Butler, in Meijer and Prins 1998: 281). Price and Shildrick (1998) also highlight the irony that people who are most visibly different often experience being overlooked, both literally and metaphorically. Disabled people are simultaneously in/visible; that is, not recognised on their terms and too visible in ableist terms. In Butler's account, Gunaratnam (2003: 48) suggests that Butler's aim is to hold out for a conceptual apparatus that will enable abjection to be thought of in different ways, to 'come out of the discursive shadows, but which does not allow it to become rigid, normative and paradigmatic'. I will turn to this point shortly when I consider thinking abjection otherwise. For now, I articulate my purposes for working with three theoretical accounts of the abject in this book: those of Butler, Kristeva, and McClintock.

I argue that Butler's notion of the abject brings a social dimension to Kristeva's psychoanalytic account of abjection, and this provides a necessary framework to explore the myriad experiences of abjection documented by the disabled people described in this book. McClintock's (1995) framework also helps to consolidate the psychic and social dimensions introduced by Kristeva and Butler. Informed by Kristeva, Butler, and McClintock (discussed in the previous chapter), I use the theory of the abject to account for the oppression of disabled lives. Disabled bodies sit outside the normative framework through which ability and humanity are constituted, and as such they are rendered unintelligible. My aim is to animate the lived experiences of abjection for the thirteen people who participated in this project (Lisa, Roger, Deb, Jake, Anne-Marie, Amal, Emma, Freddie, Joshua, Peter, Warren, Richard, and Clifton). I argue that without exploring how abjection is lived as a social process, it is impossible to explore the spaces of possibility within which abjection can be resisted and the terms of intelligibility reimagined.

Reshaping the terms of cultural intelligibility

Throughout the evolution of the project, the concept of the abject became useful in helping theorise the violence inflicted upon disabled bodies. As I continued to reflect on, refine, and apply a theorisation of abjection to the life histories of the people who participated, I came to consider the ways in which disabled people both abjectify themselves and experience abjection from others. I also became preoccupied with the question: *if certain populations are abject, are they forever abject?* While the term 'abject' historically has negative connotations, it was unclear what kind of redemptive possibilities were available to displace these destructive forces. Yet at Butler (1993: 3) suggests, abjection should not be considered as a 'permanent contestation of social norms condemned to the pathos of perpetual failure, but rather as a critical resource in the struggle to rearticulate the very terms of symbolic legitimacy and intelligibility'. To this end, my aim became to reappropriate disabled bodies from the practices in which they are culturally and socially inscribed as abject, along with the material effects of this inscription. To position disabled people in relation to the abject in this way, however, was not enough; I felt ethically and politically compelled to open up spaces of possibility where abjection can be reclaimed and resisted.

Stryker (1994) provides one example of the ways in which her own abjection has been reclaimed and embraced. When Stryker, a 'transsexual leatherdyke' (1994: 246), declares 'I am a transsexual, and therefore I am a monster', she reclaims the terms such as monster to 'dispel their ability to harm' (1994: 240). Stryker (1994: 240–241) writes:

> [h]earken unto me, fellow creatures. I who have dwelt in a form unmatched with my desire, I whose flesh has become an assemblage of incongruous anatomical parts, I who achieve the similitude of a natural body only through an unnatural process, I offer you this warning: the Nature you bedevil me with is a lie. Do not trust it to protect you from what I represent, for it is a fabrication that cloaks the groundlessness of the privilege you seek to maintain for yourself at my expense. You are as constructed as me; the same anarchic womb has birthed us both. I call upon you to investigate your nature as I have been compelled to confront mine. I challenge you to risk abjection and flourish as well as have I. Heed my words, and you may well discover the seams and sutures in yourself.

Stryker evocatively resists her own abjection and highlights how all bodies are 'constructed' in order to resist the charge that she is 'unnatural'. In this book, I open up spaces of possibility for considering how the abjection of disabled bodies might be similarly resisted, reappropriated, and reclaimed, and I return now to Butler's (1993) notion of the abject in order to consider these possibilities.

Butler's political and social abjection: changing the rules

Notwithstanding Butler's socialisation of the Kristevan (1982) theory of the abject, I am also interested in her theorisation for another, although related, concern. Lloyd (2007: 74) suggests that Butler's (1990, 1993) theorisation of abjection relies on her presupposition that 'violence is constitutive of regimes of intelligibility', and that political change is always possible within culture. Within Butler's account of the abject, then, there is the capacity of abject bodies to challenge and contest the normative violence that afflicts them. Butler (1993: 16) argues that

> it will be as important to think about how and to what end bodies are constructed as is it will be to think about how and to what end bodies are *not* constructed and, further, to ask after how bodies which fail to materialize provide the necessary 'outside', if not the necessary support, for the bodies which, in materializing the norm, qualify as bodies that matter (italics in original).

Butler (1993) presents abjection as a discursive process, where there is an 'outside' to the construction of normative bodies. Abjection, for Butler (1993: 23), is an 'enabling disruption' where the existing norms can be resisted. Butler (1993: 22) argues that abjection can provide a 'radical resignification of the symbolic domain, deviating the citational chain toward a more possible future to expand the very meaning of what counts as a valued and valuable body in the world'. Regulatory norms are sustained through reiteration, and reiteration can be resignified. Resignification can produce a reconfiguration of the hegemonic norms, such that the terms of cultural intelligibility and unintelligibility can be reshaped.

What I appreciate in Butler's (1993, in Meijer and Prins 1998) political and discursive articulation of abjection is that it is transformational. It does not heed to a pathological discourse that forever labels disabled people—or other abject beings—as abject or forever outcast in the 'shadowy regions of ontology' (Butler, in Meijer and Prins 1998: 277). As Butler (in Meijer and Prins 1998: 277) says: 'I'm enraged by the ontological claims that codes of legitimacy make on bodies in the world, and I try, when I can, to imagine against that'. Disabled people, and other abject beings, possess the performative agency within which existing regulatory norms can be subverted—or simply reinscribed. But how might this be possible? In the following section, I illuminate instances where regulatory norms have been subverted, and expose alternative notions of disabled subjectivity. Specifically, I highlight another way of re/imagining disability. While the focus of this book is concerned with unearthing experiences of abjection, my aim is to speculate about the conditions in which such acts can be resisted or reclaimed.

Reappropriation

If, as Butler argues, abjection operates at a discursive level, then discursive shifts can alter the terms of cultural intelligibility. One strategy to accomplish this has been reappropriation, which refers to the practice of embracing terms that were previously seen as jarring or derogatory. Sandahl (2003: 36) suggests the aim is to 'appropriate and rearticulate labels that the mainstream once used to silence or humiliate'. The realm of queer and feminist politics possesses several examples where once-derogatory words have been reclaimed. 'Queer' is perhaps the most well-known example; originally used as an invective against gay men and lesbians, it has been reclaimed as a term of pride, particularly for trans*[1] people who feel 'gay', 'lesbian', or 'bisexual' do not adequately capture their identity (Butler 1993; Sandahl 2003). Butler (1993) suggests that the pain caused by the 'queer' invective has actually enabled it to be/come a term of empowerment. Clare (2015: 109, italics in original) writes how 'queer' can be used as a source of pride and a defiant retort:

> [s]ometimes the words of hatred and violence can be neutralized or even turned into the words of pride. To stare down…the basher swinging the word *queer* like a baseball bat, to say 'Yeah, you're right. I'm queer…So what?' undercuts the power of those who want us dead.

The success of 'queer' reclamation has witnessed a spread to other terms, where 'dyke', 'fag', 'slut', 'whore' and, more recently, 'nasty woman' and 'cunt', have likewise been subjected to reclamation to varying degrees (Stryker 1994; Zoladz 2012). The purpose of these reappropriations is to resist the violence and political power of these words. This is not so say that these discursive shifts, which seek to destabilise hegemonic norms, entirely eradicate material acts of violence. Rather, they open ethical and political possibilities for challenging and resisting this violence.

Borrowing from queer, feminist, and race politics, some in the disability community have started to reappropriate terms. The most notable example is crip (from the pejorative term, cripple), which some disabled people have started to use to self-identify. Stella Young, an advocate and comedian in Australia, self-identified as a cripple:

> I'm a crip, and I identify pretty strongly with a crip identity. And for me, people get all up in arms when I describe myself as a crip because what they hear is the word cripple and they hear a word that you're not allowed to say anymore…I think it's important for people to understand that crip is a word I find empowering in the same way that some members of the gay community, but not all members of the gay community, find the word 'queer' empowering.
>
> (in ABC Perth Radio 2012)

Young identifies with crip for personal and political reasons, and she notes the parallels between crip and queer. Similarly, Clare (2015: 84) describes crip and queer as cousin words: 'words to shock, words to infuse with pride and self-love, words to resist internalized hatred, words to help forge a politics'. Shapiro (1993: 34) also suggests that reclaiming cripple means 'disabled people are taking the thing in their identity that scares the outside world the most and making it a cause to revel in with militant self-pride'. Important in these descriptions is the linking of reclamation with advocacy and politics; claiming crip is a political statement that can be used in everyday contexts to challenge normative practices (Sandahl 2003). It seeks to highlight conceptions of normal and abnormal, and critiques attempts to homogenise humanity.

These approaches have begun to coagulate around a new theoretical perspective: crip theory (Kafer 2013; Löfgren-Mårtenson 2013; McRuer 2006, 2011; Sandahl 2003). Largely informed by, and related to, queer theory, crip theory opposes normativity, resists the temptation to isolate its terms, substance or theoretical position, and is much more radical/provocative than disability studies (Kafer 2013; McRuer 2006).[2] One element of crip theory is cripping, which again borrows from queer theory's, queering. Queering refers to the practice of re-presenting mainstream (heteronormative/heterosexual) representations to expose queer subtexts (Butler 1993). Similarly, cripping 'spins mainstream representations or practices to reveal ablebodied assumptions and exclusionary effects' (Sandahl 2003: 37). 'To crip' means to engage in practices that challenge the oppression of normativity, and to (re)affirm disabled people's self-worth (Sandahl 2003).

One example of 'cripping' can be found in McRuer's text *Crip Theory: Cultural Signs of Queerness and Disability* (2006), where he crips the television show *Queer Eye for the Straight Guy*, imagining the hosts' denigrations of participants: 'He's so retarded!', or 'That's so mental-institution chic'. McRuer (2006) adopts Garland Thomson's (1997) definition of the normate, and proposes *a crip eye for the normate guy*. Garland Thomson (1997: 8, emphasis in original) defines the normate as

> the veiled subject position of cultural self, the figure outlined by the array of deviant others whose marked bodies shore up the normate's boundaries. The term *normate* usefully designates the social figure through which people can represent themselves as definitive human beings.

McRuer (2006: 197, italics in original) then subversively, and bitingly, proposes what a crip eye for the normate guy might look like:

> [a] crip eye for the normate guy, I propose, would not just be a disability version of the Bravo hit, no matter how much pleasure imagining such a show has given me: 'Sweetie, your university is an accessibility *nightmare*! Don't worry, honey, it is your lucky day that disabled folks

are here to tell you just what's *wrong* with this place!' Rather, a crip eye for the normate guy (and because we're talking about not a real person but a subject position, somehow 'normate guy' seems appropriate, regardless of whether he rears his able-bodied head in men or women) would mark a critically disabled capacity for recognizing and withstanding the vicissitudes of compulsory able-bodiedness.

Here McRuer (2006) crips the Fab Five's attitudes to disability, undermining ableist assumptions. The aim for McRuer is to highlight the conditions within which disabled people face oppression, and, in particular, to problematise the conditions of compulsory abledness.

Again, borrowing from queer theory, instead of the queer art of failure (Halberstam 2011), crip theory exposes the crip art of failure. In *The Queer Art of Failure* (2011), Halberstam imagines failure otherwise, and overturns the logics of success. Elias (2012: 1962) suggests Halberstam's manifesto is a

> loving tribute to those of us who fail, lose, get lost, forget, get angry, become unruly, disrupt the normative order of things, and exist and behave in the world in ways that are considered antinormative, anticapitalist, and antidisciplinary.

Failing is transformed into opportunity and opens a politics of 'solidarity, of refusal, of unbecoming and unknowing, of the absurd that all come back to failing differently, failing better, and failing collectively' (Elias 2012: 1962). Mitchell, Snyder, and Ware's (2014) work is also relevant here; in their article, they propose the active insertion of disability into childhood learning environments, or, put another way, cripping the curriculum. This, they argue, displaces the idea that disability is a failure that should be hidden, and instead advocates for interdependency rather than autonomy, and the idea that disabled people exemplify alternative experiences/expertise (Mitchell, Snyder, and Ware 2014). In a world where governments, bureaucracies, parents, and schools are obsessed with children meeting developmental, academic, and behavioural standards, disabled/disruptive children are an unreasonable presence in classrooms and playgrounds (Slater 2015). Cripping the curriculum, however, puts 'failure' on centre stage, exposing possibilities for varied forms of embodiment, ways of being, and behaviour, and promoting a shared interdependence (Mitchell, Snyder, and Ware 2014).

The notion of queer time has also spawned the concept of crip time. Halberstam (2005) speculates that the notion of queer time emerged during the AIDS epidemic, where diminished futures became a reality for many. Many queer people reoriented their focus away from longevity and futurity to focus instead on the *here* and *now* (Halberstam 2005). The saying 'live fast, die young [and leave a beautiful corpse]' comes to mind. During the release of the film *Holding the Man* (2015), an interview excerpt from Timothy Conigrave—the real-life character on whom the film is based and who died of AIDS-related complications in 1994 at 34 years of age—was released. In the excerpt, Conigrave says that because he has 'been expecting to die for so long', the idea of him ever reaching 40 years of age was a daunting impossibility. In response, 'the only thing [he] had to live for' before his death was writing a book and a play. Such attitudes in the face of the HIV-AIDS epidemic were not uncommon.

Halberstam (2005) notes that the epidemic also completely upended the conventions of family, inheritance, and child-rearing, and that the creation of alternative queer temporalities emerged from it. Such legacies continue today in similar and different forms, but for disabled people, crip time operates in a slightly different register. McDonald (n.d.) writes:

> I live by a different time to you…I have cerebral palsy, I can't walk or talk, I use an alphabet board, and I communicate at the rate of 450 words an hour compared to your 150 words in a minute—twenty times as slow. A slow world would be my heaven. I am forced to live in your world, a fast hard one. If slow rays flew from me I would be able to live in this world. I need to speed up, or you need to slow down.

McDonald (n.d.) exposes the different temporalities by which people live; yet it would be a mistake to conclude that all disabled people are simply slower, or always need more time (Kafer 2013). While some disabled people may require more time to complete certain tasks or to travel to certain locations, Kafer (2013) suggests that crip time should be about flexible time and not just extra time. Indeed, some people labelled on the autism spectrum, and some living with mental health needs, actually operate on accelerated time.

Disablist and ableist factors should also be figured in notions of crip time. For example, Kafer (2013: 26) draws upon an example of someone requiring extra time to arrive at a location, suggesting it might

> result from a slower gait, a dependency on attendants (who might themselves be running late), malfunctioning equipment (from wheelchairs to hearing aids), a bus driver who refuses to stop for a disabled passenger, or an ableist encounter with a stranger that throws one off schedule.

Crip time challenges normative assumptions about pace and scheduling, and seeks to highlight crip temporalities (Kafer 2013). Some may find crip time to be too idealistic or too incompatible with 'culture standard time' (Michalko 2010), but this assumption fails to acknowledge how time is already cripped. For example, chronic fatigue, constant pain, relapse, remission, prognosis, diagnosis, acquired, developmental, and so on are all everyday conditions or descriptions of disability and illness that are all located in time (Kafer 2013). It could also be argued that queer time is already crip time, given Halberstam's (2005) speculation that the origins of queer time lay in responses to AIDS (read: *disability*). Ultimately, whether it be queer or crip time, such musings expose the temporalities of (queer/disabled) lives, and, perhaps more importantly, how an ableist 'culture standard time' can be cripped.

Crip theory also encourages people to *come out crip*, much in the same way others have come out queer (McRuer 2006). Sandahl (2003: 27) writes that while she has never seen anyone abled claim to be crip, she would not be surprised by the practice, suggesting that 'the fluidity of both terms makes it likely that their boundaries will dissolve'. This contrasts with *coming out queer*, which is a position that is increasingly adopted by even cisgender heterosexuals. McRuer (2006: 36–37) extends this discussion by considering the reasons why *coming out crip* may be difficult:

> a nondisabled person claiming to be crip dissents from the binary division of the world into able-bodied and disabled—or, rather, affirms the collective crip dissent from that division. Since dissent requires comprehending the able-bodied/disabled binary as nonnatural and hierarchical (or cultural and political) rather than self-evident and universal, and since the vast majority of both nondisabled and disabled people have in effect consented to comprehending that binary as natural, it is in some ways not likely that anyone would claim to be crip, but most especially those who are nondisabled.

Put succinctly, the institution of ableism and the way in which disability is naturalised makes it extremely difficult for people to think around the constructions they perceive to be natural. Nevertheless, McRuer (2006: 53) highlights one example where he *came out crip*, stating, 'I came out as HIV-positive. I'm not, as far as I know, HIV-positive'. McRuer (2006: 57) writes, 'I find it more important to raise issues about what it means, for the purposes of solidarity, to come out as something you are—at least in some ways—not'. McRuer has experienced 'not insignificant periods of my adult life unsure of my serostatus' (2006: 53) and has had encounters 'where HIV was unquestionably on the other side of the condom' (2006: 57). For McRuer (2006), coming out crip enabled an examination of the politics of queer/disabled bodies. Coming out crip critiques the binary between dis/ability, 'recasts what it means to be human' (Goodley 2014: 43), and rejects the hegemony of abledness. For crip theory, keeping the terms of dis/ability open is vitally important.

Querying crip

As new theoretical perspectives enter a discipline, it is important that such contributions are fairly scrutinised. For example, some scholars have questioned the interdisciplinarity of critical disability studies/theory (Samuels 2002; Shakespeare 2013). Scholars in critical disability studies/theory often draw upon theories in races, genders and sexualities studies, and so on

(Campbell 2009; Goodley 2013; Meekosha and Shuttleworth 2009; Shildrick 2012); indeed, above I have drawn heavily on queer theory. However, Samuels (2002) cautions that substituting terms such as 'sex' and 'gender' with 'disability' risks a disturbing slippage of the terms under inquiry. Moreover, in marshalling such terms as race, sexual identity, religion, disability, and so on under one banner, Samuels (2002: 65) argues we may 'lose sight of the profound differences between these social designations'. Yet I would argue that the point is not merely to substitute terms uncritically, but to expose the points of intersection, similarity, and departure in critical terms. Critical disability studies is a relatively new academic field, and despite such critiques as Samuels (2002), I propose that its interdisciplinarity is one of its key strengths. This is because, rather than starting theoretical discussions anew, it permits scholars to borrow—where relevant—from other domains and consider disability in new ways.

Using the term 'crip' has also been criticised. Bone (2017: 1302), for example, writes that crip does not make her think of dis/ability, but rather takes her back 'to living in Albuquerque, New Mexico during the late 1980s when the Bloods lived on one end of the street and the Crips lived on the other'. For Bone (2017), crip is innately linked to gang warfare and violence, and consequently problematic to the politics of dis/ability. While I appreciate the dual meaning of this term, I am more attuned to McRuer's (2006: 65) observation that disability 'has haunted Crip reality from the beginning', where gang members are at heightened risk of becoming disabled (through injuries). Bone (2017) also suggests that 'crip' privileges physical disability while other forms of disability become invisibilised. Yet I think this argument fails to recognise Sandahl's (2003) observation that the term has stretched to include all forms of disability, and even abled people who may claim crip.

Sherry (2013), however, argues that claiming crip is available only to those most privileged, where many still find it a deeply jarring and derogatory term. He writes that in all his years communicating with disabled people, roughly 5000 of them, he can 'count on one hand the number of people who call themselves "crip" or want to be called "crip" by others' (Sherry 2013: n.p). While I appreciate this point, and Sandahl (2003: 49) reminds us not to forget that such terms 'retain the taint of their power to injure' even as we reappropriate them, I do not concede that this means we must abandon the term completely. Johnson and McRuer (2014: 247) have responded to Sherry's (2013) critique, saying it is a position they 'differ from' yet ultimately 'respect'. In response to the claim that McRuer is 'imposing…an epistemological framework' (Sherry 2013), Johnson and McRuer (2014: 248) suggest 'the work, as it unfolded, had so much to do with inviting conversation, searching out community, and wondering aloud what the word could do or mean'. In his earlier work, McRuer (2006: 40) emphasised that crip should be 'permanently and desirably contingent'. I argue that if crip is not reappropriated, it will remain a negative term. The aim should be to resist oppression, and reclaiming crip is one recourse in this aim. It should also be recognised that claiming crip is a condition of possibility (Butler 1993, 2004); not all people will claim they are crip, just as not all LGBTI people claim they are queer. It should be remembered that claiming crip is concerned with keeping open the terms of dis/ability, and of recognising the fluidity and 'leakiness' (Shildrick 1997) of bodies.

In thinking through the appropriateness and potential of the term crip, I draw on Jagose's (1996) summary of debates surrounding the (appropriate) usage of queer in the late 1980s and early 1990s. Jagose (1996) notes concerns at the time that use of the word 'queer' may actually increase the oppression and violence against queer lives, and give licence for people to come up with newer and more degrading terms. Others could never imagine politicians employing the word queer, and some simply thought it had little political value in resisting queer oppression. Nearly thirty years later, these concerns have lost their salience, including the admissibility of the term 'queer' (and 'gender queer') by politicians. This is not to say, however, that employing crip will give rise to the same level of change. My aim is merely to open, speculatively, a space of possibility within which we can begin to think differently about the terms that oppress. The status quo is unsatisfactory, and claiming crip may provide an avenue of possibility in which disabled people can re-collectivise and resist their own abjection.

However, if terms are vulnerable to reappropriation, does this apply to all terms? Are some terms off-limits? 'Nigger' is still a deeply polarising term that oppresses black minorities in spite of attempts at reappropriation. Whilst Butler, in *Excitable Speech: A Politics of the Performative* (1997)—a text considering some of these very questions—steers clear of considering this point, Galinsky et al. (2003) highlight the extent to which the aims of reappropriation between nigger and queer were very different. For queer people, the aim was to popularise the term within society, to turn the label from negative to positive and to promote inclusiveness (Galinsky et al. 2003; Jagose 1996). Yet for black people, 'nigger' was—and still is—used as a sign of affection within particular black communities, and is forbidden outside of those communities (Galinsky et al. 2003). In this sense, the intragroup privileging of 'nigger' over intergroup permissibility re-instantiates the idea that 'nigger' is off-limits, and consequently, still jarring and derogatory. The point that I take from this, then, is that the term crip cannot be confined to disabled people only. If the aim is to disarm terms of their ability to wound, creating rules about permissibility and impermissibility re-instantiates oppressive normativities. At the same time, I think it is important to recognise that those who take up terms, and are constituted by them, are best positioned to know when, how, and for what purpose, such terms are best used. It is also important that those claiming crip are invested in a politics of this sort, otherwise reappropriation risks becoming oppressive cultural appropriation. Suffice to say, this issue is much more complicated than I have given it credit for, yet it falls outside of the scope of the arguments I am making in this book (for more detailed discussions about black culture, cultural appropriation, and the politics of 'nigger', see Galinsky et al. 2003; Kennedy 2002; Rodriquez 2006; West 1993; Ziff and Rao 1997).

Reappropriating abjection?

As I contemplate the potential and merits of reappropriation, my thinking returns to the abject. Specifically, I wonder whether abjection itself can be reappropriated. Finding the work of Halperin (2007) has greatly freed my thinking on this point. In his text *What Do Gay Men Want?* (2007), Halperin reappropriates abjection in the context of gay men's lives. In reappropriating abjection, Halperin (2007) suggests that the concept can be embraced in the face of the social oppression of gay lives. He takes Warner's (1995: 35) claim that 'Abjection continues to be our dirty secret', and examines what that might look like for gay men. For Halperin (2007: 65), abjection is

> what it means to have someone's dick up our butts or to have someone come in our mouths. We need to admit our pleasure in being the lowest of the low, in being bad, in being outlaws, in betraying both our own values and those of the people around us.

If gay men are social pariahs, rather than resign themselves to this form of persecution, Halperin (2007: 65) suggests there may be a 'transgressive appeal' in being abject. Gay men are well-acquainted with 'experiences of pain, fear, rejection, humiliation, contempt, shame, brutality, disgust...[and] condemnation' (Halperin 2007: 94). Abjection for gay men may be a 'strategic response' or 'self-defense' to these experiences (Halperin 2007: 94, 92). Halperin (2007: 80) writes that abjection involves 'a bitter pleasure in humiliation', where the humiliating effects of abjection can be disarmed by depriving others of their ability to wound.

Halperin (2007) documents a scene in Genet's semi-autobiographic novel, *Miracle of the Rose* (1966 [1951]),[3] to illuminate a reappropriated view of abjection. Genet introduces the reader to a story based on an incident recounted to him about a boy named Bulkaen, whom Genet loved. This incident involved several boys tormenting Bulkaen at a reformatory. In the novelised version of this incident, Genet portrays himself as Bulkaen experiencing his torment, where he is forced to stand several yards away from the other boys with his mouth open, and the boys take turns spitting into his mouth. Initially a victim, the annihilating force of these acts begins to change, and Genet undergoes a transformation. Genet (in Halperin 2007: 76) writes,

> [i]t would have taken very little to transform this atrocious game into a chivalric one, such that instead of spit I would be covered with a shower of

roses. For inasmuch as the motions were the same, fate would not have had to go to much trouble in order to change everything: the group forms...some boys make motions of throwing...it wouldn't have cost much for the outcome to be happiness... I prayed God to ease His intention a little, to make a false movement so that the boys would no longer hate me, but love me.

As the violence escalates, Genet recounts,

I was no longer an adulteress to be stoned but an object employed in a rite of love. I desired that they would spit at me more, with thicker viscosities.

(in Halperin 2007: 76)

In this scene, abjection has been transformed from 'social humiliation into erotico-religious glorification' (Halperin 2007: 76). Genet, as Bulkaen, has transformed his fear and horror into resistance and desire. Genet assumes Bulkaen's subject position to share their abjection: 'I TAKE THE SUFFERING UPON MYSELF AND I SPEAK'.

Some may interpret this reappropriation as perverse. To be clear, abjection is neither about turning pain into pleasure nor about the joys of being violated (Halperin 2007). It is also not a pursuit for self-annihilation (Halperin 2007). Rather, abjection is concerned with finding 'unexpected opportunity' in the 'exposure to social condemnation' (Halperin 2007: 81). As Halperin (2007: 95) writes, 'the more people despise you, the less you owe them'. Abjection may actually be a solution rather than a problem, and Halperin (2007) argues that this strange paradox may be true because, after all, abjection sits at the edge of the subject. He argues that abjection 'is an experiment with the limits of both destruction and survival, social isolation and social solidarity, domination and transcendence' (Halperin 2007: 87). Embracing abjection may be an act of martyrdom in order to resist or disarm the soul-crushing effects of social oppression. But what are the ethics and politics of this account of abjection, and how might it inform an understanding of the violence experienced by disabled subjects?

Embracing abjection in the context of disability?

How do we connect this thinking to the forms of violence disabled people experience, as well as the participants who shared their stories in this book? It would be folly to presume that the participants, and disabled people more broadly, should simply embrace the symbolic and physical violence meted out to them. Rather, much in the same way reappropriation is directed towards 'words that wound' (Matsuda et al. 1993), the reappropriation of abjection should involve disarming the social injuries directed towards disabled people by reappropriating abjection as a site of contestation, survival, resistance, and self-defence. Embracing material abjection is complicated, not only because of the tangible—and perhaps even deadly—consequences. Indeed, invoking the story from the *Miracle of the Rose* (1966 [1951]), Halperin (2007: 84) notes that 'some people in Genet's situation might simply be crushed'. It is important then that we do not overly-romanticise the benefits of embracing abjection. Rather, I conceive that *embracing abjection is a transgressive and agentic act for those who choose it*. Halperin (2007: 94, italics in original) argues that abjection could be a '*strategic response to a specific social predicament*'. Further, Halperin (2007: 86–87) writes,

> abjection names the social situation that forces us, in order to survive, to resist the crushing burden of shame, to glory in our exclusion from the scene of social belonging, to transcend (at least in our imagination) the humiliating realities of social existence, and to find in the secret history of our pleasures a source of personal and collective triumph over the forces that would destroy us, then abjection would seem to have some life-enhancing uses. Abjection is not the problem, in other words, but the solution.

To reappropriate abjection means to embrace abjection, to 'relinquish the norm as a lost cause' (Campbell 2012: 226), and in so doing to deprive the current social context of its power to demean the abjected subject.

In the chapters that follow, I document various instances where the disabled people who spoke to me in my project experienced abjection. In a few examples, I expose situations where this abjection has been resisted. My aim in the preceding section has been to open up spaces of possibility where the existing status quo can be rejected. It is not enough to merely document the abjection of disabled lives; this would risk a kind of determinism, or 'poverty porn' (Beresford 2016; Runswick-Cole and Goodley 2015a, 2015b) that would situate disabled people as agent-less and forever abject. My aim, then, has been to theorise the potentiality of resisting abjection. Importantly, too, in an environment where there are a collective set of experiences inflicted upon disabled bodies, the response requires a collective set of responses from multiple agents over time and place. I return to this point at various times throughout the remaining chapters.

Conclusion

My aim in this chapter has been to introduce Butler's account of the abject and illustrate the ways in which it applies to the experiences of disabled people more broadly. Dislodging abjection from its psychic origins, I have introduced social abjection to illuminate the cultural and political contexts in which violence afflicts disabled lives. More importantly, however, I have used Butler's notion of the abject, along with queer and crip theory, to expose the conditions in which abjection might be resisted or embraced. In the remaining chapters, I share the thirteen life histories I have collected, along with my analyses of them and an account of the iterative process through which I have theorised abjection as simultaneously collective and singular, psychic and social (and see the Appendix for an overview of the ways in which the data were approached).

Notes

1 The asterisk used after trans is used to signify multiple and divergent identities that fall outside traditional gender norms, including, but not limited to, transgender, transsexual, transvestite, gender-queer, genderfluid, gender-fuck, agender, bigender, and so on.
2 Sandahl (2003) suggests that crip theory and queer theory emerged in response to the normalising tendencies of their disciplinary antecedents (that is, disability studies and gay and lesbian studies). Just as queer theory works to disrupt the normalising tendencies of gay and lesbian studies, crip theory does the same to disability studies.
3 I would have liked to reference Genet's text directly; unfortunately, I only have access to a version (1966) that is different to Halperin's translation. Comparing the translations, I believe Halperin best illuminates the concepts relevant to the abject, so I am relying on Halperin in this instance.

References

ABC Perth Radio 2012, 'Who Are You? Stella Young', accessed online 9 November 2016, <www.abc.net.au/local/audio/2012/02/29/3442495.htm>.

Beresford, P 2016, 'Presenting Welfare Reform: Poverty Porn, Telling Sad Stories or Achieving Change?', *Disability & Society*, 31(3): 421–425.

Bone, K 2017, 'Trapped behind the Glass: Crip Theory and Disability Identity', *Disability & Society*, 32(9): 1297–1314.

Butler, J 1990, *Gender Trouble: Feminism and the Subversion of Identity*, Routledge, New York and London.

Butler, J 1993, *Bodies that Matter: On the Discursive Limits of 'Sex'*, Routledge, New York and London.

Butler, J 1997, *Excitable Speech: A Politics of the Performative*, Routledge, New York and London.

Butler, J 2004, *Undoing Gender*, Routledge, London and New York.

Campbell, FK 2009, *Contours of Ableism: The Production of Disability and Abledness*, Palgrave Macmillan, London and New York.

Campbell, FK 2012, 'Stalking Ableism: Using Disability to Expose "Abled" Narcissism', in *Disability and Social Theory: New Developments and Directions*, edited by D Goodley, B Hughes, and L Davis, Palgrave Macmillan, Basingstoke, Hampshire, UK, pp. 212–230.

Clare, E 2015, *Exile and Pride: Disability, Queerness, and Liberation*, 16th anniversary edition, Duke University Press, Durham, NC and London.

Elias, L 2012, '*The Queer Art of Failure*, by J Halberstam', reviewed in *International Journal of Communication*, 6: 1962–1964.

Galinsky, AD, Hugenberg, K, Groom, C, and Bodenhausen, GV 2003, 'The Reappropriation of Stigmatizing Labels: Implications for Social Identity', in *Identity Issues in Groups*, edited by JT Polzer, Emerald Publishing, Bingley, UK, pp. 221–256.

Garland Thomson, R 1997, *Extraordinary Bodies: Figuring Physical Disability in American Culture and Literature*, Columbia University Press, New York.

Genet, J 1966, *Miracle of the Rose*, Grove Press, New York, translated by Bernard Frechtman, [originally published as *Miracle de la rose*, Librairie Gallimard, 1951].

Goodley, D 2013, 'Dis/entangling Critical Disability Studies', *Disability & Society*, 28 (5): 631–644.

Goodley, D 2014, *Dis/ability Studies: Theorising Disablism and Ableism*, Routledge, London and New York.

Gunaratnam, Y 2003, *Researching 'Race' and Ethnicity: Methods, Knowledge and Power*, SAGE Publications, London.

Halberstam, J 2005, *In a Queer Time and Place: Transgender Bodies, Subcultural Lives*, New York University Press, New York and London.

Halberstam, J 2011, *The Queer Art of Failure*, Duke University Press, Durham, NC and London.

Halperin, DM 2007, *What Do Gay Men Want? An Essay on Sex, Risk, and Subjectivity*, The University of Michigan Press, Ann Arbor, MI.

Holding the Man 2015, [DVD], Neil Armfield, Transmission Films, Australia.

Jagose, A 1996, *Queer Theory: An Introduction*, New York University Press, New York.

Johnson, ML and McRuer, R 2014, 'Introduction: Cripistemologies and the Masturbating Girl', *Journal of Literary & Cultural Disability Studies*, 8(3): 245–255.

Kafer, A 2013, *Feminist, Queer, Crip*, Indiana University Press, Bloomington, IN.

Kennedy, R 2002, *Nigger: The Strange Career of a Troublesome Word*, Vintage Books, New York.

Kristeva, J 1982, *Powers of Horror: An Essay on Abjection*, translated by LS Roudiez, Columbia University Press, New York.

Lloyd, M 2007, *Judith Butler: From Norms to Politics*, Polity Press, Cambridge, UK.

Lloyd, M 2008, 'Towards a Cultural Politics of Vulnerability: Precarious Lives and Ungrievable Deaths', in *Judith Butler's Precarious Politics: Critical Encounters*, edited by T Carver and SA Chambers, Routledge, London and New York, pp. 92–105.

Löfgren-Mårtenson, L 2013, '"Hip to Be Crip?" About Crip Theory, Sexuality and People with Intellectual Disabilities', *Sexuality and Disability*, 31(4): 413–424.

Matsuda, M, Lawrence, CR, Delgado, R, and Crenshaw, KW (eds) 1993, *Words that Wound: Critical Race Theory, Assaultive Speech and the First Amendment*, Westview Press, Boulder, CO.

McClintock, A 1995, *Imperial Leather: Race, Gender and Sexuality in the Colonial Contest*, Routledge, New York and London.

McDonald, A n.d., *Crip Time*, Anne McDonald Centre, accessed online 7 March 2017, <www.annemcdonaldcentre.org.au/crip-time>.

McRuer, R 2006, *Crip Theory: Cultural Signs of Queerness and Disability*, New York University Press, New York and London.

McRuer, R 2011, 'Disabling Sex: Notes for a Crip Theory of Sexuality', *GLQ: A Journal of Lesbian and Gay Studies*, 17(1): 107–117.

Meekosha, H and Shuttleworth, R 2009, 'What's so "Critical" about Critical Disability Studies?', *Australian Journal of Human Rights*, 15(1): 47–76.

Meijer, IC and Prins, B (with J Butler) 1998, 'How Bodies Come to Matter: An Interview with Judith Butler', *Signs: Journal of Women in Culture and Society*, 23(2): 275–286.

Michalko, R 2010, 'What's Cool about Blindness?', *Disability Studies Quarterly*, 30(3/4), <http://dsq-sds.org/article/view/1296/1332>.

Mitchell, DT, Snyder, SL, and Ware, L 2014, '"[Every] Child Left Behind": Curricular Cripistemologies and the Crip/Queer Art of Failure', *Journal of Literary & Cultural Disability Studies*, 8(3): 295–313.

Price, J and Shildrick, M 1998, 'Uncertain Thoughts on the Dis/abled Body', in *Vital Signs: Feminist Reconfigurations of the Bio/logical Body*, edited by M Shildrick and J Price, Edinburgh University Press, Edinburgh, pp. 224–249.

Rodriquez, J 2006, 'Color-Blind Ideology and the Cultural Appropriation of Hip-Hop', *Journal of Contemporary Ethnography*, 35(6): 645–668.

Runswick-Cole, K and Goodley, D 2015a, 'Disability, Austerity and Cruel Optimism in Big Society: Resistance and "The Disability Commons"', *Canadian Journal of Disability Studies*, 4(2): 162–186.

Runswick-Cole, K and Goodley, D 2015b, 'DisPovertyPorn: *Benefit Street* and the Dis/ability Paradox', *Disability & Society*, 30(4): 645–649.

Samuels, E 2002, 'Critical Divides: Judith Butler's Body Theory and the Question of Disability', *NWSA Journal*, 14(3): 58–76.

Sandahl, C 2003, 'Queering the Crip or Cripping the Queer? Intersections of Queer and Crip Identities in Solo Autobiographical Performance', *GLQ: A Journal of Lesbian and Gay Studies*, 9(1–2): 25–56.

Schein, L 2000, *Minority Rules: The Miao and the Feminine in China's Cultural Politics*, Duke University Press, Durham and London.

Shakespeare, T 2013, *Disability Rights and Wrongs Revisited*, 2nd edition, Routledge, London and New York.

Shapiro, JP 1993, *No Pity: People with Disabilities Forging a New Civil Rights Movement*, Three Rivers Press, New York.

Sherry, M 2013, 'Crip Politics? Just … No', *The Feminist Wire*, 23 November, accessed online 10 January 2017, <www.thefeministwire.com/2013/11/crip-politics-just-no/>.

Shildrick, M 1997, *Leaky Bodies and Boundaries: Feminism, Postmodernism and Bio-(ethics)*, Routledge, London and New York.

Shildrick, M 2012, 'Critical Disability Studies: Rethinking the Conventions for the Age of Postmodernity', in *Routledge Handbook of Disability Studies*, edited by N Watson, A Roulstone, and C Thomas, Routledge, London and New York, pp. 30–41.

Slater, J 2015, *Youth and Disability: A Challenge to Mr Reasonable*, Ashgate Publishing, London.

Stryker, S 1994, 'My Words to Victor Frankenstein above the Village of Chamounix: Performing Transgender Rage', *GLQ: A Journal of Lesbian and Gay Studies*, 1(3): 237–254.

Warner, M 1995, 'Unsafe: Why Gay Men Are Having Risky Sex', *The Village Voice*, January 31, pp. 33–36.

West, C 1993, *Race Matters*, Beacon Press, Boston, MA.

White, SK 1999, 'As the World Turns: Ontology and Politics in Judith Butler', *Polity*, 32(2): 155–177.

Ziff, B and Rao, PV (eds) 1997, *Borrowed Power: Essays on Cultural Appropriation*, Rutgers University Press, New Brunswick, NJ.

Zoladz, L 2012, 'A Fascinating History of the "C Word"', *Alternet*, 14 August, accessed online 14 August 2017, <www.alternet.org/gender/fascinating-history-c-word>.

3 Deb's narrative

Exploring the multi-dimensional forms of abjection

Deb lives a normal everyday life, and her life is just like those of the other participants in this research—and, I would suggest, most people reading this book. She enjoys time alone, but has a network of familial, social, and professional relationships that keep her active. Her experiences are unique, yet simultaneously collectively produced and constituted. My aim in this book is to provide a multi-dimensional account of abjection, and in this chapter, I use the life history narrative of Deb to begin and build this account. My aim is to foreground the different dimensions of Deb's abjection using McClintock (1995), Kristeva (1982), and Butler's (1993, in Meijer and Prins 1998) theorisations. I illuminate how the various dimensions of abjection described by McClintock—objects, states, zones, agents, groups, and psychic and social/political processes—come together in particular temporal and spatial contexts, and examine how abjection is distributed, cyclical, compounding, and often invisible. My aim is to make visible the ways in which disabled bodies are violated and regulated, and how abjection works on Deb's body to produce a particular type of disabled subject. Importantly, however, in tracing Deb's narrative, I also focus on the sites of struggle that she employed to resist her own abjection.

In exposing the multi-dimensional and iterative nature of Deb's abjection in this life history, I also seek to foreground the (crip) temporality with which she conveyed her storytelling. This means I have made some strategic choices to present Deb's story in a particular way. First, while I have chosen to speak *about* the participants, I am also simultaneously trying to foreground the participants' own narratives. My aim is to make a clear distinction between *my* voice and *Deb's* voice. I foreground both Deb's voice and my voice throughout this chapter, sharing the storytelling in different parts and at different moments. Second, and relatedly, when presenting Deb's narrative, I have chosen to share unedited excerpts from the transcripts, as I want to maintain veracity to her words and the rhythms of her speech. I want to maintain integrity to the ways in which she—and all of us—communicate verbally, including intonations, contradictions, false starts, stuttering, and so on. Specifically, I seek to illuminate the (crip) temporality with which she spoke. Third, the sequence of the story I present characterises the sequence in which Deb told her story. When I first met her, Deb spoke almost non-stop for forty minutes about a vast array of experiences. She mentioned names and places to me as if I already knew them, and jumped from story to story without any clear indication of how they related. There was no distinct chronology to the stories, and many stories were sparse on information and self-reflection. However, during subsequent interviews, we constructed a more coherent narrative, and in this chapter I maintain integrity to the crip (and cyclic) temporality with which she delivered these narratives.

In making these decisions, parts of the story below may seem chaotic. I ask the reader for patience and perseverance. It will be emotionally demanding (particularly given Deb's stories of abjection), but it is important that we stay as close as possible to Deb's mode of storytelling. To replace contradiction with consistency, ambiguity with clarity, and chaos with order would commit a form of symbolic violence against Deb. I am also reminded of Spivak's (in Danius and Jonsson 1993: 33, italics in original) assertion that '*plain prose cheats*',[1] and that, according to Butler (1999), the rules of grammar constrain thought. I want us to privilege the crip temporality with which Deb speaks, and arguably, to demand coherence in a text *may* itself constitute a form of ableism (Goodley 2014).

The day I met Deb

In my first interview with Deb, I knew very little about her and was unprepared for the traumatic story that was about to unfold. My first question invited her to tell me a little about herself, and she spoke almost non-stop for the next forty minutes:

> Um, my name's Deb. Um, I was, um, put away into institutions from under six months old, 'cause I had epileptic fits … And from six months to five years old I went to a home called XXXX … but there were things that happened to me like, the good things I remember was the nu-, um, the priest, I used to steal his food, 'cause he got better food than what the children got there, and that. And I used to go through the window and steal, steal his food, before he got back, before he got there … And, I can remember when you used to wet the bed, if you wet the bed the nuns of a morning, 'cause the beds were all, all in a row, they were, but there was that much of a gap [indicates about a foot] for the nuns to walk down, they would feel each bed of a morning, every morning this happened, and if you've wet the bed, and there was other children that did the same thing, and if they've wet the bed and I've wet the bed, they'll go 'right, you get back into bed'. And they'll get the sheet, put the sheet right over your head with the real big safety pins and pin it to the pillow, and you had to lie underneath that sheet in the wet of your urine for an hour. And sometimes you'd go without brekky, and that was to make the nuns teach us a lesson, that would, yeah. But when you were little,

you don't, you can't teach them a lesson 'cause it happened to me a hell of a lot, you know I was only a little girl, I was. And I remember the boiled lollies we used to get … I can remember when we used to go for our walks as well of a night time with the nuns, and we used to go around the lake, with the nuns. Mm. Which I remember. And while I was there I was always a problem child, too, because I didn't know, 'cause of my fits, they used to call me monkey word, they did … called me monkey too, is because my skin was so brown, and me, I didn't know then that I was indigenous … I was a problem child all the time, and I was always in trouble, and that, and it was to do with the fits, which I didn't know then 'cause I was so young … always in trouble, I was a problem child, and that's why they called me monkey, and that, and even probably 'cause of the skin, too, and I was so brown.

Deb's epileptic fits have constituted her as abject within a society that pathologises and marginalises difference. Her medicalised/pathologised embodiment requires that she be removed from the public and institutionalised, ultimately compounding her abjection. Within the zone of this institution (which I will provocatively call the 'asylum' [Goffman 1961] from now on), Deb is shaped by the practices through which her body is violated and regulated. Being forced to lay in wet urine (a process of abjection) is a debasing and dehumanising act (Sherry 2010), and it reminds me of Shakespeare's (1994) description that disabled people are constituted as 'dustbins for disavowal'. Deb has already started to document the ways in which her abjection is compounded, how it entraps her, and how she is situated within a double bind. For example, because Deb is abject she is deprived of food; if she chooses to steal food she becomes abjected again as a thief (as a 'problem child' and (brown) 'monkey'). Deb's abjection is thus established as a transaction which she must use to negotiate the world; she has the agency to resist or relent, but she must face the consequences. The asylum and church represent two intersecting institutions that work to abjectify and regulate Deb, working together to discipline and punish (Foucault 1977). Punishment works as a regulation of the norm, yet Deb understands that her punishment is unjust and unfair. Wetting the bed is often involuntary (just like occupying a socially abjected group), yet Deb is punished regardless.

Deb then started talking about her move to another institution:

And then after that, from the age of five I went in the car with a nun, and that because they were waiting for a vacancy from one of the institutions … and the institution that came up vacant … was not so pleasant. I was there from the age of five until 21. Um, at five I was in a ward … and that was five to 10. And there was some things that happened there, like I can remember the wet grass, and we had to sit on that wet grass, and we used to get rashes, and we never had cream for it or anything, for that crea-, for that, you know, the rashes. And, um, that was sore for a while, you know, for a couple of weeks or whatever, because of sitting on the wet grass, and that, and it was not right, to me it wasn't. And then, um, I can remember Charlie the Strap, as well. Um, when you were in the institution you would get Charlie the Strap across your legs, across your ass, across your back, across your arms, you know. And even if you swore at the staff, as well, or back-chatted, you would get the strap again. And that. And you would even go to bed early at five o'clock, that night.

Deb's reference to a 'ward' hints to the medicalised world she has entered; she is a patient in a ward, not a child in a home. Deb cannot comprehend the violence inflicted upon her; in her mind it is unfair, but for the institutional agents it is discipline used to constitute and regulate the abject disabled subject. Her body is regulated; abjection is distributed throughout parts of her body (legs, ass, back, arms, and mouth), where they become abject objects through contact with 'Charlie the Strap'. The children are constituted as inferior to the staff, and they are governed according to regulatory norms where children must listen to adults and 'speak only when spoken to'.

Immediately after the dialogue above, Deb progressed to another incident:

And I can remember that there was a place … [a]nd there woulda been about, I'd say about 82 or, 80 kids that never had families to go to, and there used to be 10 staff who used to come along with us. And of a night time there was always one staff that looked after about 80 kids while the other staff were up at the pub enjoying themselves, having a drink and tea, talking and all this, while we had to stay down there … And one of the staff that was on night, on night duty that night, um, I was only six and I wanted to go to bed early, and he said to me 'you do me, you do me a big favour first', and I go 'what?' He goes 'you rub my head for an hour', so I rubbed his head but I was still falling off to sleep, and then I said to him 'can I go to bed' and he goes 'I'll take you up to bed, I will', and he did but he touch, touched me, down below, touched me on the boobs, he played around with me, and then he watched me get undressed too, and then he took me down to the toilet, and then he pulled his pants down, and that, and hanged it out, and I had to touch it. I didn't know what it was, and he played around with me again, and watched me on the toilet, when I was, going to the toilet. And he knew I was close to [the Johnson's],[2] he did. And he said to me not to tell anybody, or I'll not be able to see [the Johnson's] again, so I didn't. And that happened to me at the age of six years old.

Deb continued:

But the funny part was, when I went back to, to the dump, to the gaol, I went up to the boys' ward in a couple of weeks down the track … 'cause I thought it was ordinary thing, and I got into serious trouble then.

This is the first of several experiences of sexual assault that Deb would recount. This experience exposes the relations of power operating within the asylum, through which agents of abjection (priests, nuns, adults) are able to mobilise their power, and power to abject, within the zones in which they work. Deb must also navigate her own abjection; she is afraid during the event, and she is also scared of the future because her relationship with the Johnson's may be deprived. Deb is abjected by the agent who violates her, yet if Deb tells anyone her abjection is compounded by being constituted as a victim, a liar, a troublemaker, or, in some ways, promiscuous (recent research has also shown that black girls are sexualised at an earlier age than white girls, see Epstein, Blake, and González 2017). She is in a difficult situation and feels that she has little possibility to do anything; she is abject no matter what. The agent of her abjection has also treated Deb like a sexual object, which constructs her as a dehumanised subject (Carlson 2010). This was also echoed in *Warren Goodwin's* narrative, where a nurse in residential care made Warren 'feel [his] big cock', degrading Warren as an object of the agent's own sexual gratification. At the time of the interviews, Deb also called the asylum a 'gaol' (comparative to 'ward' earlier), indicating she perceived herself as an inmate in the zone of a prison rather than a resident in a home. In the second excerpt of the above narrative, we can also see how this sexualised behaviour has become normalised for Deb, such that she went into the boys' ward and thought it was an ordinary thing. In this sense, we can see how her abjection has been compounded again—her experience of sexual violence has been normalised, such that she thinks sexual practices are normal in the asylum, and gets into trouble (abjected) again for being 'promiscuous' with the boys from the other ward.

Deb then told me that at 10 years of age, she was moved to another ward in the asylum with about thirty-five to forty other girls. She mentions:

> we had to polish the floors and mop the floors and that, and that was every morning we had to do that, and we would get into trouble from the school for being late to class … we used to have our boyfriends we used to go under the pipes, and kiss, hug, and that, I remember … we used to have sports days as well, and I used to be a fast runner … And the parents used to come up, I mean not my parents but other people's parents who was in the institution as well.

Here, Deb documents her relationship between multiple institutions: the asylum, her school, and (absence of) family. Deb again cites the double bind she is in; if she does not mop the floors adequately at the asylum, she is punished, yet if she mops them too well, she is punished at school for being late. Deb is punished for transgressing in a context where the boundaries are opaque and shifting, and this form of symbolic violence gives occasion for physical violence. Deb also mentions how she lacks a significant part of most people's lives: a family.

Deb immediately started documenting another story:

> And, um, I can remember at the age of 13, like the [other ward], they used to go swimming a lot on the weekends, but, um, one particular staff member would not let us go. And the … girls did want to go swimming, and I said to 'em 'do you dare me, if I go down the front office?' and they go 'oh yeah, I dare ya'. So I said 'alright, I'll go down there'. So I went down to the front office and I told the big boss, and I said 'all the other wards are going swimming and the boss in our ward will not let us go swimming, so can you ring them up, ring her up and tell her?' He goes 'first, do me a big favour, first. Get in the other office, pull your pants down, get yourself ready, and then I'll lock the front door'. So he locked the front door and he came into the other office, 'cause there were other offices there down in the front office, and he pulled his pants down and he got hanky ready, and he asked me to wank him until it came. And he played around with my fanny, my boobs, you know, touched them, and had a good play around. And then when that was finished he said to me 'right, don't you ever [emphasis] tell anybody, because if you do, you're not gonna go swimming again on a Saturday when I'm in the office'. So I didn't tell anybody. And we went swimming.

Another staff member has sexually abused Deb, and like the previous story, her punishment and abjection is constructed as a bargaining transaction that she must use to negotiate. Deb wants to go swimming; this is a sign of her advocacy, resistance, and agency, yet this is punished by the agents of her abjection. To go swimming, Deb must be subjected to sexual violence. Her abjection is compounded; she occupies a socially abjected group, yet is victim to the processes of abjection and further confined to an abject zone (the office) within an abject zone (asylum). Zones and agents distribute her abjection. And again, if she allows the violence she is abject, but if she reports the conduct she is abjected again, whether as a victim, liar, or so on. Slowly but surely, her conduct is more tightly regulated and agency limited through the distribution of her abjection. The various dimensions of abjection are entwined at different times to keep her in her place.

Deb then moved on to this story:

> and then I can remember on a Sunday, when one particular bus driver used to take us to church, and he got attached to some of the senior girls, but he also got attached to me. And he said 'would you like to come out, you know, on day trips with us, with our family?' and I go 'yeah'. He goes 'I'll talk to the family, then I'll find out from the front office if we can'. So they got the permission to finally say it was OK, so I went out with the family, and of an, of a Sunday after he took us to church, I used to stay on the bus and put the bus away with him. Um, with the bus company, you know … And when he used to do that, it

didn't happen straight away but down the track he said to me, because it st-, he started touching me first through the clothes, and then down the track under the clothes, and then down the track he said to me 'go out the back in the bus and get yourself ready, and pull your pants down and wait for me'. So I had to do that. And he said, then, um, close the gate, the main gate of where the bus company is. And then he pulled his pants down, and then he got his condom out and put it on, and then he raped me. And I didn't know this but I was only 16 then. And I said to him 'why am I bleeding?' He goes 'you've got your period', and I go 'ohhh'. And then he said 'don't ever tell anybody what's going on between you and I, or the family, or you'll not go out with us again'. And that went on for three years, in the back of the bus. That did. And, I didn't tell anybody, until like, um, I think about five, six years ago. I, I remember, um, one of the ladies who I must of told from the hostel, but I told her not to tell anybody. I told her to keep it to herself. You know, 'cause she remembers from when I told her. But, um, I used to even work in their shop as well, and of a night time this was on a Friday and a Saturday morning, and of a night time, on a Friday night, he would call to say to the family 'go home, it be only Deb and I here', we'll go down to, there's, there was a stairway, and he used to keep the, you know, the food down there, and he used to come down and he raped me, down there, too. Um, in the shop. And then after that, that happened for three years down there as well. Um, because see me I used to think I was being free when I was going out with them, and I used to have good times with them, but I had the bad times as well.

The dimensions of abjection are forever shifting for Deb, exposing the temporal and spatial factors that mediate her situation. Her abjection by the bus driver has become ritualised, where the behaviour escalates over time to see how she responds. Sexual penetration is a process that fully and literally violates the insides of the body. Yet Deb has the agency and awareness to choose how she responds to this situation. She knows that inside the asylum, she is abject, and while she is still abject on the outside, at least she has the opportunity to be 'free', have fun with others, and enjoy human connections.

Even though Deb is caught in a continuous cycle of sexual violation/abjection, she tolerates it because she is on the outside. In this sense, abjection does not work top-down from agent to abject; the abject also have the performative agency to resist various dimensions depending on the context. To be sure, this behaviour does not absolve the sexual violator of their conduct, and it should not be assumed that Deb is choosing between a good or bad option. Both options are bad; she just needs to choose something that gives her a viable life. For Deb, the possibility of her 'freedom' on the outside is contingent on her (sexual) abjection by the bus driver.

Deb moves on to another form of sexual violation:

> And I remember the walks we used to go on as well, we used to go on long walks up the back of, of the dump, the gaol ... We had to hold ourselves, but if we wet ourselves, we had our nose rubbed in it.

Sherry (2010: 12) suggests the presence of urine during violent acts is a symbol of sexual domination, where the intent is to 'dehumanize, objectify, violate and sexually degrade the victim'. These actions again show how the children's bodies are regulated, where urination on long walks is prohibited. If they do urinate, they are punished with their noses rubbed in it. This is a degrading and debasing process of abjection, reminiscent of how animals (dogs, particularly) are punished if they commit the same act.[3] This demonstrates how the disabled subjects in the asylum are constituted and dehumanised if they do not conform to regulatory norms. Deb's references to 'the dump' and 'the gaol' also illustrate her relationship to the asylum today.

While in the asylum Deb also learned how to crochet:

> I used to put it in the ... [local] Show, um, you know and I used to always win, 'cause I was in with the special school. But one time I remember I told one of the teacher's 'I want to go on the outside, not on the inside, and I want to have a go on the outside', but what he did, she do, she put it on the inside with all of us, when we're called 'retards', 'spastics', 'mental case' and all that, in those days.

Deb is presented here with a fissure between what she knows of herself—and her advanced skills to master crochet—and what the world thinks they know of her. Notwithstanding the violence in the zone of the asylum, here is an illustration of public violence where those at the local show call Deb and the other children 'retards', 'spastics', and 'mental case'. This form of violence was also echoed in *Richard Brady, Amal Alam, Clifton Murphy,* and *Warren Goodwin's* stories, where disablist abuse was directed at them in public settings because of their non-normative subjectivities. Not only is Deb subjected to violence and regulation within the asylum, she experiences this from outsiders. This operates as a symbolic marker for where she (does not) belong in society as abject, and illustrates how her abjection is distributed. Yet even though Deb experiences abuse from others on the 'outside', she desires to be on the outside because it is a normative place to be, and preferable to the inside where she is sexually violated (even though she believes she can negotiate the circumstances of this violence). Disabled/abject bodies are often told they fail to reach the norm, yet to displace this oppression, many try to be as normal as possible.

Deb immediately moved to another story:

> Yes, and with, and while I think of it I'm gonna jump the gun and go from one extreme to another extreme, and this is to do with violence,

this is. When I was living … with the ex, and happened about 3 years ago, or, yeah, and, um, my ex was violent to me 'cause of, um, my epileptic fits. 'Cause while I was having the fits I was too scared to go to people, I was. And, um, when, I used to always be scared of him 'cause he had a violent, because of his father, 'cause his father was violent as well. And I used to be scared, because of people wouldn't help me, 'cause of those days in the institution when people didn't help you, and then that was while I was having the fits.

Deb commenced this section of the narrative by mentioning that this story was different to the previous because it focussed on violence; perhaps Deb does not conceptualise the previous event (discrimination and verbal abuse) to be violence, and this perception is particularly common amongst disabled people (Thorneycroft and Asquith 2015; Williams 1993). For many disabled people, violence can become so normalised that they no longer perceive themselves to be victims (Thorneycroft and Asquith 2015; Williams 1993). At the time of the sexual assaults, Deb also did not perceive herself to be a victim, constructing it as an 'ordinary thing'. In any event, Deb has now documented three different abject zones in which her body has been regulated and violated: numerous events in the asylum, the local show, and in her home from her ex-partner, David.[4]

Each incident re-instantiates her abject status, normalises the violence, and institutionalises her abjection and 'abnormality'. Deb cites two explanations for David's violence: her fits, and because he inherited his violent streak from his father. This is the second occasion Deb has identified her epilepsy as the state that causes the violence against her. Deb also implicitly documents the effects of the asylum, and how this has affected her behaviour and emotions outside the institution. Deb was too scared to go to people and get help for the cyclical and repetitive nature of her abjection from David because in the institutional days, 'people didn't help you'. This also illustrates that the staff's role was not to help the children, but rather to regulate and punish them as abject bodies. They are constituted as abject subjects who have few options to escape violence.

Deb told me that she met David through his brother, Adrian.[5] Adrian was also a resident at the asylum. Below, Deb describes how her relationship with David changed after her surgery:

I started to stand up, and be, and that, 'cause I had brain surgery in 2004, and, um, that's when I started to be more independent, and I didn't need him, and he didn't like that. And you know, when we had our last fight, a couple of years ago, 'cause I kept going to Melbourne and all this, getting involved in organisations and that, and, um, on our last, on our last fight, this was when he kept me hostage in the community house, after I had the brain surgery, and I was scared of him, I was. But, um, he threatened me and he headlocked me, slapped me across the face, and he was banging doors in and out all the time, he was trying to throw things at me, 'cause he never had his medication, I never had my medication, 'cause he's got a lot more health problems than I, what had, about seven of them ... I was scared of him but I was so used to the fights that we were having, and I was not upset, and I had to at the end of the day, 'cause it was all night he kept me hostage, I had to that morning try and cry, which I did try and cry.

While she was in a scared state, the abuse from David became entirely normalised for Deb, such that she was 'so used to the fights' that she was 'not upset'. Perhaps Deb is desensitised to her own abjection. Yet on another level, she knows it is wrong, and she forced herself to cry after the event. She also locates the cause of her new-found independence as her surgery that has cured her epilepsy. After the surgery, Deb said she was more independent and no longer needed him, and in doing so, resisted and reoriented the existing power dynamics in the relationship to try to break free from the cycle of abjection. Psychology and medicine have pathologised Deb; yet paradoxically, medical intervention has offered her the freedom from her abjection and the restoration of her humanity. Deb also must abject her epilepsy in order to (re)affirm her identity and integrity (Kristeva 1982).

On the day Deb left David, she went to the police station to report the domestic violence. And now,

since I'm in, living in Melbourne I am free's a bird, and I love it! Yes, and because me being indigenous, this is for the indigenous people too, the violence. 'Cause they get violent, a, they have a lot of violence going on them too. And even when they were in these institutions, they were sexually abused, physical abuse and all that, too! You know, yes. Hmm.

Deb recognises that disabled and indigenous people are inequitably victimised. This is an implicit acknowledgement of her new-found, multi-layered identity, and a recognition that she belongs to two oppressed minority groups.[6] She specifies she is now 'free', occupying a non-abject zone in Melbourne. Yet it is also interesting how her construction of freedom is contextual and shifting. For example, previously Deb said she felt free, but this was while she was being raped outside of the asylum. For Deb, she was free because she was outside the asylum, suspending (momentarily) the various compounding forms of her abjection and its intensity. Various dimensions of abjection work at different times and in different places, such that today she is still abject (as an 'intellectually disabled' subject). However, various dimensions of Deb's abjection have dissipated or been re-framed through processes of resistance, such that her freedom takes on another form in another zone.

Deb's monologue ended at this point. I was shocked, floundering, and did not know what question to ask next. For some unknown reason, the one thing left lingering in my mind was family (or more accurately, the absence of family):

> (So did you see your family at all while you were …)
>   No because at the age of eight, when I was in the institution, before eight I thought the institution was my family. But once I turned, when I turned eight in the dining room they got some information from down the front office and, they said 'oh Deb, we've got some information for you down the front office your mum's dead, do you know that?' They didn't care. They were just there for their job and money, the staff were. Yeah. And I didn't eat all my tea that night, and I remember the nurse who took me to the … ward, and I was still not eat my tea, and then that night when I went to bed I was still crying, and one of the nurses who was on night duty that night punished me and told me to shut my mouth, stop crying, or I'd go up to the, um, thing, and I did, 'cause I kept crying. On my knees against the wall with my hands on my head, my head. For an hour. Mm.

Deb recounts how she was punished for engaging in an entirely normative practice: grieving. In the asylum, children are trained to have no emotional responses; they must be quiet to have a viable life in an asylum, otherwise they are punished. Deb's abjection is again compounded; not only is she in a state of grief, she is punished for engaging in this process of grieving. The state of grief has no place in the asylum, and we can see how Deb had to unlearn the practice and 'try and cry' when David assaulted her. Her abjection means that she is punished for acting normally—grieving—when she is constantly constructed as being not-normal. This puts considerable weight on Deb to unlearn and relearn certain practices and behaviours, and how certain behaviours are normal or abnormal within different temporal and spatial contexts.

Deb's story about her mother's death was yet another shock for me. Then I asked, 'So, what was, can you remember the good times?'. In hindsight, I completely minimised everything Deb had told me with this question. I think this is indicative of my inexperience with fieldwork at the time—this was my fifth interview out of forty-five. My explanation at the time was that I was shocked at what Deb had told me, and in efforts to escape the trauma I asked for 'good times' to help me process what had just been disclosed. I also think my confidence and competence evolved throughout the interviews. Overtime, Deb and I built greater rapport, and I endeavoured to avoid abjecting her through reducing her to a research object. Rather than ask questions and simply expect answers, I learnt to be a witness to the violence and be *in the moment* of Deb's narrative.

When I asked Deb why she thought the staff treated her and others badly, she replied:

> Because they thought, in those days, they thought that we were retarded, spastic, mental case, and they thought we never had a voice, in those

days. They thought that since we never had a voice, that they'd be able to get away with it. But today, they don't, they can't. But, 'cause people are telling their stories and what happened in those days.[7] And they, they're on the losing end but we are on the winning end.

Deb illustrates how disabled people are produced as abject bodies within the asylum, as bodies that do not matter and are voiceless. Deb also invokes a binary logic between winning and losing; previously she was on the losing end, but now that those things have changed she now perceives herself on the winning end. She also highlights the historical dimension to this violence. Decades ago this was the norm, whereas today there are other iterations and practices—often invisible—that marginalise and oppress disabled people. Years ago they could get away with physical and sexual violence, yet today this is not uniformly the case. Decades ago disabled people in asylums lacked the necessary agency and this made them 'losers', but now that many disabled people are deploying their agentic force by coming forward to tell their stories; for Deb, this makes them 'winners'.

I asked Deb how the bullying and abuse made her feel. She said,

Oh yeah definitely, I was scared, frightened, I was only a little girl, you know. Like, people wouldn't believe ya, they would think that you were talking out of your ass, they would think. Know what I mean? Mm. They would think that you were making it up.

Deb identifies how (disabled) youth are subjected to suspicion when they report wrongful behaviour. Young (disabled) people are often constructed as untrustworthy and unbelievable, and so Deb's abjection is compounded as both a child and a disabled subject. Deb was scared, but she had no one to talk to about the violence.

Deb also spoke more about her ex-partner David:

Um, I was, I was too scared to go to people, and he would, he would always be the boss, the domineering person, and I would always be the chook, you know, being, being scared, and that. And, um, you know, I wasn't allowed to say anything, I just had to keep that mouth shut. And that, that was while I was having fits a lot, and all that because it was still, I was still staying back in the past, but once I had the fits, once I had the brain surgery that's when things changed and he didn't like it at all. I was starting to be more independent, going to Melbourne a lot more, him doing the housework and all this, which he didn't like, he wanted me to be at home, and I didn't want that, you know. So he was on the losing end 'cause I left him for violence, for domestic violence, and I was on the winning end. It's like these three men that did it to me, I'm on the winning end now, and they're on the losing end. And they are dead, they are under the ground, they are. With the, um, with the, um, ghosts. Yes.

David employs multiple processes of abjection against Deb—various forms of physical and emotional violence. It is also interesting that Deb compares herself to an animal—a scared chook. Deb describes how she was in a state of fear, illustrating how endemic it is to her own abjection. In addition to her disabled identity, there are gendered dynamics waged between Deb and David. David had expectations about the relationship: Deb must be submissive and he dominant; Deb must do housework while he does not; Deb cannot talk while he can; Deb cannot leave the house but he can. Deb must also keep her mouth shut, like her days in the asylum. Deb continues the binary logic, saying she is today a winner and not a loser. Again, Deb has cited her epilepsy as the cause of the violence and abjection. Once her epilepsy is cured, however, the dynamics between them began to change, and this altered the relationship between them. Her stand against David is also a surrogate for standing up against the three other men who sexually violated her.

It was somewhere at this point that our conversation had gone for about an hour, and it was time to conclude. I recall going to the airport for my flight back to Sydney, and I felt sad and alone. Here is an excerpt from my research diary:

13/7/2015

Met Deb and interviewed her … I was lost for words. I didn't know what to say. I didn't know what topic[s] to follow up. In hindsight I really floundered for the last half hour. I just, I couldn't do it. At the hour mark I just wrapped up the interview. I can't recall what we discussed in the second half [of the interview], I was just stunned and didn't know what to say. After the interview Deb and I hugged each other. She really touched me. I need to be mindful of this …

The first interview with Deb affected me greatly, such that my diary entry simultaneously says so little yet conveys a great deal. My lack of voice and ability to process what Deb told me found its way into my diary entry. Upon reflection, my interaction with Deb raises an important question: *is abjection contagious?* If we accept that abjection, in its etymological sense, means to 'cast out', Deb may be expelling on to me her own abjection. I am interested in an intersubjective exchange of the psychic and the embodied dimensions of abjection, such that I experienced them as my own. To preserve her own subjectivity, she needs to recount her stories to others, perhaps to me. And what did I do with this abjection? I took it up, accepting her abjection inside me. I then called my mother at the airport; perhaps moving the abjection onwards to her. In this sense, abjection is shared and relational, both a singular and collective experience, and perhaps partly voluntary and capable of resistance (Halperin 2007). As I spoke to my mother, I drank beer in the airport lounge, wanting my brain to turn numb. Abjection makes us vulnerable, so it is important we have the interdependency to turn to others (or perhaps *anything*). The distributed, compounding, and iterative nature of the practices of abjection requires mechanisms to eschew its power.

Interviews two, three, and four—building on what came before

In subsequent interviews Deb and I expanded the content that was covered in the first. For example, in later interviews I learned that she was 54 years old, loved looking through old photos, and was very protective of her independence.

Previously, I have speculated how various dimensions have worked to violate and regulate Deb. In the first interview, she focussed largely on the zones and agents in the asylum, abuse at the local show, and the domestic violence she experienced. I subsequently learned of more family violence, albeit in a different form. Deb learned through her institutional records that her mum 'neglected' her. Deb's mum was a 'prostitute'[8] who smoked marijuana and drank alcohol while pregnant. Deb says she was

> unfed, kept dirty on the mat, on the bed, in the nuddie, howling my eyes out. Um, sometimes I'd be in the cupboard, close the door. You know, locked up in the cupboard, howling my eyes out.

When Deb's mum was ready to work, they would both go to the local pub, and Deb was placed on top of the bar. Deb was having epileptic fits at the time, and Deb explains her mum 'lost bond with me'. Here, Deb is abjected through abandonment. Eventually the courts decided Deb would be placed in an asylum.

In our second interview, we spoke about Deb's experience of sexual abuse and rape. Deb reflected on the sexual abuse she experienced when she was 6 years old:

> I just didn't know. I was just too scared, and I wasn't, I was just too scared to say something, frightened, very frightened, at the age of six. And that's why, and I had fits too, and I didn't know what was right, what was wrong. You know, I just thought it was an ordinary thing, what he was doing. I thought he was allowed to do that, at the age of six, but I didn't know. I wasn't taught that.

Deb says she did not know what was right or wrong, and she considered the sexual abuse as an ordinary thing. Her abjection has become ordinary and expected. This reveals the extent to which subjects are regulated within the zone of the asylum and told or not told certain things about the norms outside the asylum. This links back to Deb's comment that 'before eight [years old] I thought the institution was my family', and that anything outside of the asylum is 'freedom'. The zone of the asylum works with its own sets of rules and standards, and this permeates to all its members, even staff. When Deb is not educated about topics surrounding sex and consent, she is not equipped to deal with such incidents. The secrecy imposed upon the children spreads to the staff, where they have their own rules, behaviours, and secrets that are withheld. The abjection, the secrets, the fears, and the punishment are distributed differently, and often invisibly, throughout the asylum according to the various flows of privilege and power between staff and children.

I asked Deb whether she would go to the police today should something happen to her again:

> Now I would, yeah, but back in those days you couldn't. But it won't happen to me again, I know it won't.
> (Yep)
> Yeah. 'Cause [Adrian], who's in [a location], he, he tried to get sex out of me, and when I left [David], I told sister don't give that phone number of mine to him, and don't give the address to him. Because if he finds out I'll go to the police.

Today Deb has the agency to go to the police if something like this happened to her again, and she also cites historical shifts that make complaint-making easier in contemporary times. At the time, however, Deb did not know what to do, or who to trust.

Deb's reference to Adrian above confused me, so I asked her to qualify it. She told me that Adrian raped her repeatedly after she left the asylum:

> he was getting sex out of me once I moved into my own unit. And he was forcing himself onto me 'cause I'm the one that had to buy the condoms. And it was even going to the footy as well, coming back to the footy. He would go down a hill for a bit where there's those toilets and he would get sex out of me there, too.

In this narrative, Deb has highlighted her lack of agency where the offender is able to get what he wants without her consent on a cyclical basis. While she has moved from the abjected zone of the asylum and the agents who have abjectified her, other zones and agents have taken their place, and similar processes of abjection continued for much of her adult life. The conversation progressed:

> (OK. So when you say that [he] was forcing himself upon you ...)
> Yes?
> (Would you, would you classify that as, as very similar to the three other men?)

Yes.

(Yep, so you would …)

I was scared, you know? It was rape. You might as well say like [rapist's name], when I was raped by [rapist's name] at the age of 16.

I asked Deb how long this went on for, and she replied:

This? Oh, well I, like, this went on for ages with me, with [Adrian]. Because I was in the flat for about two years or whatever. But even before that, when I was in the CRU,[9] I used to go down and visit him but he didn't, he always used to touch me and that, but he used to not try and get sex out of me, but with other people. Do you know what I mean? And he waited for me to live on my own.

(OK. Yeah. Um, and so why do you think he was targeting you?)

'Cause I was an easy target because of my disability and epilepsy, and because of my upbringing in the institution when people would never believe you. He thought that he can get what he wanted and he did. And, um, people would not believe me, um, if I told them or if I did tell them. You know what I mean? They'll just think I'm making it up.

Again, we see a continuation of the logic Deb has previously stated where people in the asylum would not be believed. Abject people have no credibility because they are dehumanised. This has also been indoctrinated into Deb at an early age, and from her life history, we can trace the way it has influenced her decision-making into adulthood. Adrian raped her for a two-year period, and Deb felt she could not do anything about it to stop this cycle of abjection. Deb said he stopped raping her when she started seeing Adrian's brother, David. As Deb says above, when she moved to a new house, she made sure that Adrian would not know how to get in contact with her.

When Deb was asked about the men who sexually abused and raped her in the asylum, she replied:

Well people who did it to me are all dead. But, uh, thing is, I've done my case, but these people, these men, three men, or might as well say two men, who did it to me, have done it to other boys from that same institution, and that's why that fits my story, on what the lawyers told me, because back before my days, when I was in the institution, they did it to those boys, before my days. And that's why it fits the story of mine.

Deb has told her story to the *Australian Royal Commission into Institutional Responses to Child Sexual Abuse*. While to some people Deb's story may seem too unbelievable to be true, her story is believed within the specific institutional setting of the commission. Deb also mentions how these sexual violators have distributed abjection widely, with many other bodies violated.

Deb also said that she told someone else about her experiences when she was in the asylum and told them not to tell anyone. This person did not tell anyone until many years later when she told lawyers associated with the Royal Commission that she recalled the conversation with Deb. I asked Deb why she thought these men targeted her, and she replied:

> They went, I reckon because they went for me, because I was an, uh, slow person, a retarded person in those days, and epilepsy, and they, they took, uh, easy chance to get to me, which they did. And they knew that I was scared, and they, when I, when I was scared, they knew they were winning, and that's why they did it.

Deb cites 'disability'—and her epilepsy in particular—as the reason for the men's violence. The institutional conditions also gave rise to the opportunity for the violence to occur, where asylums are filled with locked doors, private rooms, secrets, and codes of silence (Goffman 1961). According to McClintock (1995), abjection works with multiple dimensions, meaning any and all parts work (or do not) in different ways, times, and intensities. Disabled people have been constructed as deficient and without agency within these asylums. Deb understands that she has been made abject and as someone who was free to be violated by those who desired it. She invokes the winning/losing binary again, recognising the offenders were winners and she was a loser. The offenders thought Deb was an easy target, and her state of fear motivated their crimes.

Given all the terrible things that happened to Deb, I could not help but ask her how she healed from it all. She replied:

> Oh. I try and move on and, um, try and get people who are not put into these institutions to learn, a, listen, you know, get them to hear what these people had to put up, so if they ever have kids, or if they got a family, not for them to do it to their children, so they won't be sexually abused. But see, sometimes I reckon, see the staff that did it to me, I reckon that it was their families probably that did it to them.
>
> (OK)
>
> Its followed in the genes, and that does happen, you know what I mean?

Deb draws on a genetic discourse to speculate about the offenders' motivations, suggesting previous victims turn into offenders. Deb may have acquired this discourse from the asylum, where their focus is on medicalisation, diagnosis, and cure. The hegemony of psychological disciplines within the asylum may have influenced Deb to draw upon medical understandings to explain the violence inflicted upon her. She may have also drawn upon this discourse to divest the individual and society from blame, such that the offenders could not help but commit the violence. In this sense, perhaps Deb is also abjecting them as a way of casting off their violence, and constituting herself as a random victim and not a deliberate target. In any event, Deb says she likes to tell other people about her experiences to help her deal with them.

When Deb was older, she was placed in a house with other girls adjacent to the asylum. Staff came and checked on them occasionally. When it came time for Deb to leave the asylum at 21 years, she went to stay in a community residential unit, or a group home. She recalls being very scared, but liked that she had more freedom. Obviously the asylum regulated her conduct almost completely, and the prospect of greater agency also daunted her. Deb got a job as a domestic cleaner at the local hospital. The job itself is reminiscent of the asylum, where she continues to mop floors and clean bathrooms. The message seems to be: *know your place in society, Deb.* This message is further embedded when she is bullied relentlessly. Deb explains,

> I got hell all the time from the staff up there, because I was one of the clients from an institution that was retarded, and that's what they looked at me on.

She also said,

> They were very mean to me because they knew that I was from the institution. And just because I was from an institution, they always treated me different. They did. Yeah.

Her abjection in a previous zone (asylum) has followed her to a new one (hospital), albeit with new agents and new processes of abjection. Deb was overworked. Asked how it felt, Deb replied, 'I felt horrible, I felt like I was always being picked on, and I was scared a lot, you know'. In this part of her narrative, we can see how the abjection of Deb in the asylum has compounded her abjection in another context: the hospital workplace. In each of these examples of violence—in the asylum, in her family, in her relationships with David and Adrian, at the local show and the workplace—we can see how Deb has been marginalised and regulated as a disabled subject. Her abjection has become normalised. It is also possible to see in explicit terms how her abjection is being reproduced from one abjectifying context to the next. Deb is abject in the asylum, and this influences how she will be treated in the workplace. She is not just a cleaner, worker, or employee; she is a 'retard' from the asylum. Deb is stuck in a perpetual cycle of abjection. One question I consider is, 'how does she change the contexts that reproduce her abjection?'

Resistance

After leaving the disabled asylum, Deb stayed and worked in the town for about five years. When Deb met David, she quit her job. From one institutional space to another, the violence merely took on alternative forms, from verbal abuse in the workplace to physical and emotional assaults in the home. Around this time Deb discovered her sister wanted to meet her, so she and David decided to move back to Melbourne in 1989, when she was 26 years old.

Deb and David lived in Melbourne together, and while it was good at the start, he became violent after about five years of being together. Deb was still having fits on a routine basis, so she found it difficult to leave. Further, Deb says,

> Because I was so used to it because of the institutional days, that they wouldn't help you, they wouldn't believe you. But that's why I didn't go to people, because of those days.

The legacies of the asylum endured, where violence becomes normalised and expected. Deb said the violence she experienced from David was physical and emotional. Asked why she thought he did this to her, Deb replied:

> 'cause he had, his father was domineering, and his father was a violent person, and so was he ... they all followed in the genes ... he would throw things, punch a hole in the wall, I had to work out how to say sorry to him in a certain way.

Again, Deb draws on a genetic discourse when she locates genes as the cause of David's violence. Deb describes David as 'the king of the house, you might as well say'. Interestingly, Deb also talks about navigating the processes of her abjection, negotiating with David as she did with her three other sexual violators. Deb says she 'put up with that from when I was 26 until 41, I did, 'cause that's when I had the surgery'. Deb is referencing the brain surgery she had in 2004, which cured her epileptic fits. The surgery lasted for five hours, and part of her brain was removed.

Following brain surgery, Deb documents the emergence of her independence:

> You might as well say the egg, and then the yolk running out, and that was saying that I was starting to stand up for myself, to be as free as a bird.

Deb has re-introduced an animal metaphor; where earlier she was a scared chook, she has now transformed into a free bird. Deb has transformed the ways in which she was previously regulated and subjected by the various institutions she engaged with and the agents operating within them. She also suggests how she changed her own behaviour with regard to these issues. Deb said she 'was still scared of him, but get more confidence'.

Deb started to go to places on her own, leaving David alone and often with housework, which he did not like. While her increased independence was beneficial, it also brought greater risk. Deb explains, he started to see the change in me, and he did not like that, 'cause I was taking away his domineering, I was. And the more I went out, I would not be happy at home. I would always, he would be the one that be doing the washing and all that, and I be out. 'Cause I didn't want to stay around, I really didn't want to stay with him, but I was too scared at the time, but once I started to get my confidence up more, started to get stronger, we had our first fight, gave him a chance, then the second fight a couple of years down the track, gave him one more chance, third fight, I said, 'cause the second fight we had I told people, in 2006, around what's going on.

(Yep)

And that's when people started realising what I was doing. But this third fight, the final fight, just a couple of years ago, I left him, for good. 'Cause the second fight, I wanted them to go back and tell him, to warn him, but they mustn't of. Or they, if they did he didn't listen.

(Mhm)

So that third fight, I left. I couldn't take it anymore, what I was, what happened to me when I was having the fits, and even when I was, had the brain surgery, I just couldn't take it anymore. Had a guts full of it. So now, I'm not interested in guys, I'm just gonna be on my own for the rest of my life, 'cause I'm glad I left at the age of 50, that's the half way mark of your age, of when you live. And from 50 onwards it's gonna be as free as a bird, 'cause you only live once on this Earth, and that's how I see it.

How Deb chose to give David three chances is reminiscent of the transactions she undertook as a victim of sexual violence in the asylum. If she does not tell anyone about her rape in the asylum, she receives a benefit, and all these years later, if David continues to beat her, she will take away a reward and inflict a punishment by leaving him. She also hints how she started to resist against David, pointing to her power and agency.

In the above narrative, Deb has also split her life in two; the first fifty years were terrible, but the next fifty will be better. Her abjection has been produced and reproduced through all of the institutional frameworks she has encountered. Yet curing her epilepsy, and learning of her sister and indigeneity, provided the opportunity to break free from that abjection. In the face of a history of abjection, Deb has made a viable life for herself once freed from the epileptic fits that she articulated as central to her abjection. It is also fortunate that Deb found new subject positions, including her indigeneity, that she did not perceive to be abject. I asked Deb if she ever saw David again, and she replied, 'Nah, he's dead'. When she left him, Deb went to the police station to report domestic violence. She also gathered up her possessions, and she moved to a new place on her own where she still resides today.

In spite of the trauma Deb experienced, she is very much an optimistic person. Whenever I saw her, she would give me a big hug, and she was always enthusiastic. Yet before each interview, she would take a tablet to help calm the nerves; evidently, her experiences are still difficult for her to recount. While there are many negative experiences in Deb's history, she looks back fondly on other events as well. Looking back, Deb was happiest when she left the asylum ('the dump/gaol'), left David, and found out about her indigeneity in 2009. Deb went back to visit the asylum a couple of years ago, and there were some rooms she could not go into because of bad memories. She has no plans to return, because 'that was enough'.

At our second interview, Deb mentioned that her life and personality could have been different if several things had not happened to her. I asked her to reflect on that, and she said,

> Well, I'm like, I'm seeing it, like how my life is now is good, like, because my life now is good, but, in one way, not to talk about the sexually abuse way, but in the other ways like the physical abuse, it's taught me a lesson to stand up for myself, to have a voice, to be heard, not to be scared of people, to not domineer people, um, because I'm really strong now, but if I was never put into a home I would have been weak. In other words, I would have had people try and boss me around, tell me what to do. And I can't, I don't do that now, because my institution, because of the stuff, being hard on us and touch on us, and the hard things we went through, that's why I'm tough.
>
> (Support worker: mm)
>
> You know, now. Yeah, but I would have been different if I wasn't put in an institution, I would have been a soft person. I'm a soft person but I'm talking about people take advantage, still. Like today, if I hadn't had the surgery. But now, I don't, 'cause of my upbringing in the institution, it was hard and tough, and that's how I am in my life.

While Deb's experiences have certainly been regulated by the various institutions she has engaged—the asylum, family and relationship networks, and the public sphere—and these have shaped her experiences and behaviours, I could not help but feel saddened that Deb thought she would be a weak or soft person had she not experienced the terrible things she did. Ultimately, this aligns to a discourse within dis/ability culture that says that disabled people constantly need to 'overcome' things in life to become as fully human as possible (Titchkosky 2007). Where does this assumption leave the abject body? That they must suffer to be strong? Yet perhaps Deb is simply finding a strategy to rationalise the behaviour she experienced and live a viable life for herself. Yet again she subscribes to a binary logic between tough/weak and hard/soft, conceptualising them as opposite and incompatible. In a later interview she reflected more:

> Well, if my life could be different, I would, I would want to, um, I would not, I would have wanted to not meet him, meet [David], if my life was different now. And I would have wanted to meet someone else, who was nicer, generous to me, kind to me. An indigenous guy I would

have wanted to have met. And I would have wanted to have kids with him, if I never had the, if I never had fits, in those days. If I had the surgery in the 20s, in my, when I was 20s, in my 20s, I wouldn't have even gone with [David], would have gone with someone else.

Deb was dependent on David due to her epilepsy, and she imagines things would have been different if epilepsy had never been part of her life. In this sense, Deb abjectifies her epilepsy.

Since Deb separated from David, her life has been much better. She loves painting and crocheting. She has many photos, and she likes to put them into photo albums. Deb goes to several disability organisations when she wants to socialise; evidently, aspects of familiarity inherent to institutional life are still part of *being Deb*. Otherwise, she enjoys living her life all on her own now. As Deb said several times throughout our conversations, '[a]nd now I'm free as a bird'.

Considering Deb's story

For most of Deb's life, her abjection has been normalised. Each institutional zone and the agents within them have regulated and violated her. While the form of violence differed from one institutional space to another, it was merely another iteration of the same workings of abjection. Yet there was a turning point in Deb's life that has led to a reclamation and resistance of her abjection. The curing of her epilepsy, discovering her sister, and learning about her indigeneity all assemble to enable Deb to create her own viable life. I argue that the animal metaphors she used were not accidental. She started as a scared chook but transformed into a sailing bird. For the yolk to run free (as she previously described), the shell must break. Perhaps the shell breaking is a metaphor for her skull being opened, her epilepsy cured, and a viable life being foreseeable. Deb is now, as she says, as free as a bird.

We can read from Deb's story much about the multi-dimensional aspects of abjection. But perhaps more importantly, her story has exposed those spaces in which abjection can be resisted. It is telling that indigeneity is also abjected, but for Deb this belonging liberates her from her (disablist) abjection. In order to free herself from abjection, Deb also needed to abjectify epilepsy. Deb's life is epitomised by a cyclical experience of abjection, but one from which she was eventually able to break-free. One question that arises from this, and which I turn to in the next chapter, is this: can someone similarly break-free from their abjection if their abjection is characterised not for its cyclical nature, but by its chaos and fragmentation?

Notes

1 I recognise that Spivak (1993) is addressing the charge that her language is too impenetrable, but I think that this point also works in reverse (that clear and simple language falsely reduces the complexity of meaning). This also reminds me

of Law's (2004) work, where he seeks to highlight the 'mess' and contradiction of meaning, experience, method, knowledge, and so on.
2   Not their real name.
3   There is a linking here with Douglas (1966: 36) definition that dirt is 'matter out of place'. The regular place for a child to urinate is inside (and a dog, outside); if they perform the opposite they are constituted as 'dirty' and must be subjected to punishment.
4   Not his real name.
5   Not his real name.
6   Interestingly, she does not mention her gender.
7   Deb is referencing the *Australian Royal Commission into Institutional Responses to Child Sexual Abuse*.
8   My preferred nomenclature is sex worker, but I have used prostitute because this is the terminology Deb used.
9   CRU stands for community residential unit, and they are group homes that house disabled people.

References

Butler, J 1999, *Gender Trouble: Feminism and the Subversion of Identity*, 10th anniversary edition, Routledge, New York and London.

Carlson, L 2010, *The Faces of Intellectual Disability: Philosophical Reflections*, Indiana University Press, Bloomington and Indianapolis.

Danius, S, Jonsson, S, and Spivak, GC 1993, 'An Interview with Gayatri Chakravorty Spivak', *Boundary 2: An International Journal of Literature and Culture*, 20(2): 24–50.

Douglas, M 1966, *Purity and Danger: An Analysis of Concepts of Pollution and Taboo*, Routledge & Kegan Paul, London.

Epstein, R, Blake, JJ, and González, T 2017, *Girlhood Interrupted: The Erasure of Black Girls' Childhood*, The Georgetown Law Center on Poverty and Inequality, Washington, DC.

Foucault, M 1977, *Discipline and Punish: The Birth of the Prison*, Vintage Books, New York.

Goffman, E 1961, *Asylums: Essays on the Social Situation of Mental Patients and Other Inmates*, Penguin Books, Middlesex, England.

Goodley, D 2014, *Dis/ability Studies: Theorising Disablism and Ableism*, Routledge, London and New York.

Halperin, DM 2007, *What Do Gay Men Want? An Essay on Sex, Risk, and Subjectivity*, The University of Michigan Press, Ann Arbor, MI.

Kristeva, J 1982, *Powers of Horror: An Essay on Abjection*, translated by LS Roudiez, Columbia University Press, New York.

Law, J 2004, *After Method: Mess in Social Science Research*, Routledge, New York.

McClintock, A 1995, *Imperial Leather: Race, Gender and Sexuality in the Colonial Contest*, Routledge, New York and London.

Meijer, IC and Prins, B (with J Butler) 1998, 'How Bodies Come to Matter: An Interview with Judith Butler', *Signs: Journal of Women in Culture and Society*, 23(2): 275–286.

Shakespeare, T 1994, 'Cultural Representation of Disabled People: Dustbins for Disavowal?', *Disability & Society*, 9(3): 283–299.

Sherry, M 2010, *Disability Hate Crimes: Does Anyone Really Hate Disabled People?* Ashgate Publishing, Farnham, Surrey.

Thorneycroft, R and Asquith, NL 2015, 'The Dark Figure of Disablist Violence', *The Howard Journal of Criminal Justice*, 54(5): 489–507.

Titchkosky, T 2007, *Reading and Writing Disability Differently: The Textured Life of Embodiment*, University of Toronto Press, Toronto.

Williams, C 1993, 'Vulnerable Victims? A Current Awareness of the Victimisation of People with Learning Disabilities', *Disability & Society*, 8(2): 161–172.

4 Roger's narrative
Abjection amidst chaos and fragmentation

Whereas Deb's life history reveals a repetitive cycle of abjection, and finally a rupture from that abjection, Roger's life can be characterised by fragmentation, opacity, and uncertainty. While Deb's crip time is circular, Roger's is fragmented, and in this chapter I illustrate how the various dimensions of abjection assemble(d) to constitute Roger and his experience. Unlike Deb—who was at times able to mediate the circumstances of her abjection—Roger alienated himself (self-abjection) and saw everyone as an agent of his abjection. Violence and anger are central to Roger's narrative. In this chapter I contrast Roger's experiences of abjection with Deb's in order to illuminate how similar and distinct forms of abjection can result in dis/similar experiences and outcomes in certain spatial/temporal contexts. I also foreground McClintock's (1995) seven dimensions of abjection (objects, states, zones, agents, groups, and psychic and social/political processes) in examining Roger's life history narrative.

In constructing Roger's life history narrative, I have presented it in a slightly different way to Deb's. In the previous chapter, I foregrounded Deb's authorial voice by quoting extensively from her transcript and making a clear distinction between her voice and my theorisations. However, with Roger these distinctions are not so easily made. For Roger, chaotic movement and contradiction characterise his story *and* his mode of storytelling. He spoke constantly, yet repetitively and ambiguously, often moving away rather than towards detail and clarity. Thus, if I worked with Roger's transcript as I did Deb's, I would risk giving an account of his life history that was largely unintelligible, which further silences rather than broadcasts his experiences. Consequently, I have summarised certain material by taking different information from different interviews and sections of the transcripts and putting them together in a more coherent form. While Plummer (2001) suggests this is an inevitable practice, I do this to pragmatically help make Roger's life history accessible for the reader. I consider this less than ideal as it increases my own intrusion into the retelling of Roger's narrative. Simultaneously, I also maintain the chaotic nature in which Roger told his stories in order to both respect and represent his own crip time. Further, I have inserted my own responses into Roger's crip time through italicised text that responds to what is opaque in Roger's narrative.

Roger Cobb is 67 years old, and most of his youth was spent in and out of asylums. Roger lives in Melbourne, and at our first interview, I learned he was in a relationship with *Lisa Austin*, another participant in this research. Roger describes himself as someone who has been hard-done-by, and who has always had to fight because he has been treated so poorly. Roger's life can be characterised by chaos, movement, contradiction, fragmentation, and uncertainty. He often spoke in generalities rather than specifics; it was as if he had so many thoughts at once that he often struggled to articulate any one coherently. As will become clear for the reader, it seemed that Roger struggled to make sense of his life and how he ended up in certain situations. At the end of our last interview together, I asked Roger if we missed anything from his story, and he replied:

I think the only thing they [the reader] might find missing is: 'why didn't that person get the support he needed?'

In Roger's account, he has been abjected his entire life and recognises he is abject. *What kind of support did Roger have? And what kind of support did Roger want, or need? And what support might have helped him?*

Roger was born in England in 1950. He was the sole child of a single mother, and even before his twelfth birthday, he was being abjected by the state and those around him. He explains,

I remember going to see, I don't know what you call them, whatever you call them, psychiatrists, psychologists, or, whatever you want to call them, I like to call them the nut factory. But, um, I remember him, he was giving me these pictures, it might be a drawing or something and you have to tell him what you see in that drawing, and then, which I thought was absolutely stupid but never mind. And then you had to put these round, these blocks in the, in the squares, you know where the, the square or triangle, whatever. And, uh, I got half way through with that and thought this is ridiculous, stupid, and I just threw the thing and walked out.

This anecdote illustrates the hegemony of psy-disciplines in defining disabled lives at the time (which still occurs today), where Roger is being tested to gauge his 'normality', or more specifically, his departure from the norm. Various dimensions of abjection are present in Roger's description; he is in the abject zone of a psychologist's office, and the psychologist is an agent of abjection who seeks to place Roger in a socially abjected group (as disabled, as a retard). The normalising gaze of psy-disciplines constitutes Roger's abjection. Implicit in Roger's story is that he was constituted as non-normative, such that he must be tested and treated, regulated, and normalised. Warner (1999: 53) writes,

[n]early everyone, it seems, wants to be normal. And who can blame them, if the alternative is being abnormal, or deviant, or not being one of the rest of us? Put in those terms, there doesn't seem to be a choice at all.

'Normal' works as a 'discursive organizer'[1] (Davis 2013: 1) and a benchmark against which all people are measured. Many disabled people will try to be normal, and most will certainly fail, sometimes. Constituted as abject, Roger is also in an unwinnable position that compounds his abjection. If he performs the psychologist's test, he possibly fails to be diagnosed as normal, and if he resists doing the test, he fails anyway, and so is doubly abjected. This is mirrored in Deb's narrative where if she is sexually violated, she is abject, and if she resists or tells someone, is still abject. This exposes the multiple and changing double binds that entrap abject bodies across shifting temporal and spatial contexts. Like Deb, Roger is stuck in an abject subject position, and in response to this, he acts out with anger and violence.

Roger describes himself as being a 'bugger of a kid' but not worse than most others. He was always outside playing with his mates, and he loved primary school. When his grandparents died, Roger travelled by boat to Australia with his mum on the advice of her sister, suggesting it would be a better life for the both of them. On the ship something happened to Roger, and the way in which he described it, and made sense of it, represents a broader pattern throughout his life and his mode of storytelling:

Anyway we were on board that, and I remember nice warm days, and I used to sit near the pool. Anyway this stupid idiot came along picked me up and threw me in the pool. And just before he went through I said 'I can't swim, I can't swim!' 'Too bad you're gunna learn', and he threw me. And someone must of heard me, and of course they came and rescued me, and uh, that person was um, I don't know, I think they locked him up somewhere until they got to a port so the police could handle it. Um, I don't know much about that, but that was that.

Who was the man? Why did he do it? Why was he arrested? Did he try to drown him? What happened to him? These are questions that Roger cannot answer, and as the reader will come to learn, Roger frequently told stories about his experiences that he struggled to make sense of, perhaps because they were not his stories but stories told to him.

Roger and his mother arrived in Port Melbourne to meet his aunty, uncle, and cousin. Roger describes them:

as soon as I met my aunty and uncle I knew I didn't like them. I hated them. I don't know why, I don't know what it was they'd done. I don't know if they done anything to me when I was back home in England when they lived there, I just knew that I hated them. And I knew that we weren't gonna get on.

It is a recurrent theme in Roger's life that he did not like certain people when he first met them. Roger understands the abject state he is in; perhaps he thinks people will not like him, so he takes a position of agency and dislikes/abjects them first. He perceives his aunty and uncle as agents of abjection, and he tries to resist his own abjection by abjecting them first.

Roger went to live in country Victoria with his aunty, uncle, cousin, and mother, and he was put into a primary school where he started having problems. Eventually,

> I had to go see another psych, what I call a psychiatrist, I don't know what you call them. Here in Melbourne. Again the same thing, blocks and pictures and whatnot, and, uh, he was saying to me on the second trip, 'instead of you coming down all this way, and having to spend all that money, your mother having to take time off work, how would you like to go into a boys' home?'[2]

The cause of the psychiatrist's evaluation is unknown, yet Roger leapt at the opportunity to enter the boys' home because he wanted to escape his extended family.

Roger stayed in the zone of the boys' home between 12 and 17 years of age. He enjoyed the experience and was particularly fond of the cottage parents. He also got on well with the other kids. He struggled with schooling and at one point was kept down a year. In a later interview, Roger was asked to clarify how he ended up in the boys' home. Like his experience on the boat, he does not know. Opacity and fragmentation characterise many of the stories Roger told me, and given the hedging he often performed when recounting stories,[3] I often thought he was trying to hide something from me. *Perhaps he does not know the answer? Perhaps he just does not want to tell me?* Today Roger relies on his memories, old institutional files, and Google searches to help him construct his narratives. Yet Roger approaches these investigations tentatively. He has the ability to access all of his files from the asylums through a freedom of information request, but he only has a few files. The topic of getting more files was raised between Roger and his support worker:

> (Support worker: You know if you get your file through freedom of information, that might tell you ...)

> I've got my file through, when I was in the boys' home, but the, when XXXX was reading that to me, there was a part in there that really shocked me and I didn't like.

(Support worker: So you don't want to get the [other files], just thinking …)

Well.

(Support worker: might answer that question, but then it might upset you as well, so.)

Well, I'm, I'm, I'm often thinking whether, whether I want to do that because, [3 second pause] it can't be any worse than what I found with, with, with my other file. Um, but I wouldn't, I wouldn't want to do it by myself so I'd ask someone like you or somebody if you'd be there with me, to read it.

Roger is caught in a predicament; he simultaneously wants to know but is scared of what he might find. Perhaps this is partly why Roger conveys stories in a fractured manner. He recounts things he only partially recalls or cannot remember, or he only recalls certain parts. There is a tension between things being fragmented, him trying to put them together, and the fear of doing so.

From the information he does have, and can remember, Roger said that he

was reading somewhere about, that my aunty was wanting to do, get a psych assessment done on me, because she thought I was cuckoo. [Pause] I was a, I was a violent boy, no more violent than, than any normal teenager, but yeah.

On another occasion he said,

that's one thing I've wondered, because one of the things that, with, I think I googling a while about XXXX boys' home and how you ended up there, and it's for parents who can't cope with their children, or are at risk, the children are at risk from, from, from their parents.

As far as Roger is concerned, his family and the psychologist are agents who conspired against him. Roger's aunty thinks he is non-normative and best regulated through psychological intervention and his placement in the abject zone of a boys' home. In response to his abjection, Roger employs violence, yet he does not see it as violence, or at least no more violent than normal. In this sense, Roger is (possibly) normalising the violence he commits in efforts to normalise his own subjectivity. *What does this then mean for Roger to experience violence from others?*

The events after this are somewhat fragmented, but it appears Roger was sent to a training farm[4] at 17 years of age. The purposes of the training farm, and the reasons for his move there, again remain unclear. He got there by cab, and upon arrival, once I got out of that cab I knew I'm not gonna like this place. I don't like the people, I don't like the manager, I don't like anybody. My intuitions were right again. Why? Because of the way I was treated, the way I was abused, the way I was manhandled, um, the way I was sexually assaulted, um, you want me keep going?

Roger recognises the agents have the power to abject him (like his aunty and uncle did), and this expectation is another form of abjection. It may be that his intuitions come from knowing that he is in an abject zone, where he reads micro-expressions and behaviours as signs of danger. In any event, his prescience of doom was correct. Roger stayed at the training farm for no longer than two months, and there were several distressing events that happened to him during that short time of 'incarceration'. One incident involved the installation of post holes, where two young men coaxed Roger into assessing the depth of the hole. The two young men

grabbed hold of me legs, stuck me head first in, in, in, in the hole, split my legs wide apart and just grabbed me really hard. You can imagine where they grabbed me. Of course I'm yelling and screaming.

Roger told the man in charge of the training farm, who he variously called 'landlord' or 'manager', but the man did not care. Roger describes the act they committed as sexual. He says,

When I say sexually, I don't mean, uh, what I'm trying to say is that I was touched in inappropriate, inappropriate places. I was grabbed in inappropriate places. That's what I mean by sexual.

Roger was asked why he thought he may have been targeted, and he said,

I don't know, maybe because they see me as different. Maybe they, maybe they, um, maybe they thought I was a bit cuckoo, or a bit slow, or bit backward, or, even though I didn't think that, I didn't think that.

Like Deb, Roger uses the metaphor of a bird—cuckoo—and it is a metaphor for madness. Even at such a young age, Roger is developing the idea from others that he is perceived differently, and that this difference is negative. Even though Roger did not think he was different, each abject zone has re-instantiated the idea in his mind. There is a circulation of discourses that congeal as the truth of Roger's self: that he is (negatively) different and abject.

On another occasion Roger accidentally sliced his finger while mowing the lawns, and he was beaten for it by the landlord/manager:

he hit from the top of my shoulders, right down to the bottom of my ankles. I was black and blue all over.

Like Deb's story of 'Charlie the Strap', Roger's whole body becomes a zone and object of abjection. Roger tried to run away from the training farm twice, but agents of abjection—police officers—returned him both times. Upon his return Roger was threatened with a ball and chain, but he cannot recall with certainty whether this happened. Whether this was fantastical or real, this memory is symbolic of the extent of his abjection, of his sense of being a convict. He is moved constantly, yet he is simultaneously stuck. He says,

> Throughout my life, we've been having to fight for things, and I'm still fighting now in 2015. I was fighting in 1962 when I didn't want to leave England, but I was too young I had no say, I had to leave, you know, that was that, you know me mum said 'right, we're going, end of story'.

Various dimensions of abjection have iteratively worked to violate and regulate Roger's conduct and location, re-instantiating his abjection and highlighting his lack of place in society. As he said,

> on the training farm, you know, I felt unloved, unwanted, I felt alone. I felt like I was alone, like a hermit.

Roger felt alone with his mum, his extended family, the boy's home (to an extent), and now in the training farm. Isolation is inherent to abjection. Eventually the landlord/manager feared for Roger's safety, so he was returned to the boys' home.

Roger was too old to be placed in the boys' home, so he was located in a room adjacent to it. Again, Roger is constantly moving through zones in which he never quite belongs. Soon after, he went into supportive accommodation, and he did not like it there either. Roger moved again, but this place was worse:

> Absolutely hated that place. Hated it with a passion. And all you'd sit and do all day was putting screws together, or putting paste together, and sticking labels on something. I don't know, what the crap is this.

This is a common response from Roger; he is frustrated and in a state and zone of abjection. Subjecting disabled people to rudimentary and repetitive tasks operates to render them into the abject state of a docile body: a body that may be 'subjected, used, transformed and improved' (Foucault 1977: 136). According to this logic, disabled people are perceived as useless, so disciplining them with 'correct training' (Foucault 1977: 170) works to constitute them as efficient and productive in a society that does not see them as either (even if they do not see the purpose for the activities they are performing).[5]

In any event, after this, Roger went to yet another new place. It was difficult to ascertain how or why Roger moved from place to place, and like before, there is a tension between Roger wanting and not-wanting to know the reasons for his movements. His predicament also points to the ways in which the asylum and its agents have regulated Roger's movements, limited his agency, and provided no/little information to him, thus fragmenting his capacity to account for key life events. His account is similar to Deb (discussed in the previous chapter) and *Richard Brady's*, who were also institutionalised in an asylum. Unlike Deb and Roger, however, Richard did not want to talk to me about his time in the asylum, telling me,

> I try to forget what happened in the past, you see. I worry about what's happening now, and the future.

Deb, Roger, and Richard had no say where they went, and no information was provided to them. To be abject is to be subject to others' authority and ambitions, and to have one's capacity for agency and sense of stability diminished. While Deb has been able to follow the movements of her abjection and its cyclical nature, Roger's movements are chaotic and fragmented, and he struggles to make sense of them.

After leaving the last asylum (and again it is unclear how this happened), Roger ended up on the street. He was about 19 years old at this point, and sometimes he used to sleep at a refuge for 'drunks'. Around this time something happened to Roger that he does not like to talk about, and the hedging he performs when communicating is again illustrated. In our first interview, he said this:

> Um, anyway something happened in, in, in, afterwards, um, uh. Police was involved, um, I ended up in the police station, um, uh, they made me sign a statement, asked me if I'm willing to sign the statement, I said 'yes'. I was absolutely petrified. Wasn't, didn't have a clue what in the hell what was going on, didn't know anything about rights in that, in those days. Didn't know anything about speaking up. Anyway I, I signed all these papers that they asked me to sign and um, when I went to court, uh, the judge, I ended up in, uh, [prison] for a while, in remand, and ended up getting in a fight there.

Roger says he knew nothing about rights, because, after all, they had been taken away from him long before. The asylum regulates Roger's behaviour, telling him what to do and when to eat and sleep; this practice is so normalised that Roger's agency and awareness of rights is limited. He draws on a contemporary rights discourse that comes from the disability self-advocacy movement (that Roger is currently involved in), where there is now a large focus on the rights of disabled people. He now understands the abject position he was then in, and that there are now mechanisms—self-advocacy—that can be mobilised to address those inequalities. *But what was the 'something' that happened? Why was he before a judge?*

Roger went on to say that the judge sentenced him to two years' probation on the condition he sought psychiatric help, so Roger signed himself into another asylum. The hegemony of psy-disciplines means that Roger's agency and freedom have simultaneously been taken away from him and (re)tied to incarceration and cure. He is forced to seek psychiatric help (as a condition of his freedom), and this confirms and compounds his abjection. Given the ways in which Roger's mode of narrating his experiences leapt from story to story, and because I did not wish to interrupt its unfolding, I was not able to address the ambiguity in the narrative above (*what happened to make him come before a court?*). In our second interview, he touched on the court case briefly, and in the third interview, I broached the topic with him again:

> OK, so what would you like to talk about?
>
> (Um, so, if any of this is too sensitive then just let me know too, but I know we've kind of touched on briefly the events about before you went to [prison])
>
> Yeah.
>
> (Can you talk a little bit more about that?)

Roger then held up the yellow sign, indicating he wanted to skip to the next question.[6] The interview progressed:

> (Next question. OK. Can you at least tell me about, um, your time in [prison], like how long you were there and stuff?)
>
> I was there for about a month. I was in remand and then I, I ended up in the hospital part, basically for my own protection.
>
> (Yep, so was that from, say, other prisoners?)
>
> Uh no just from the, uh, the time when I, uh, I hit the other resident, the other prisoner, sorry.

It is telling that Roger says 'resident' before correcting himself with 'prisoner'. Institutional spaces are endemic to Roger's life, and he conceives each to be similar. So too, Deb described herself as living in a gaol. That Roger conflates asylums and prisons speaks volumes to the ways in which disabled people are regulated like prisoners.

The conversation continued:

> (Yep, so it seems like there's, like, a bit of a trend about trying to keep you safe in all the institutions, from the other people and perhaps the

people in charge, and all that kind of stuff. So how did, how was your relationship with these people like?)

[Pause] Um, [pause] I couldn't understand some of them, you know, uh, basically, uh, basically I thought they were my friend, but, um, uh, [pause] yeah. A couple of times I ended up in the locked ward, and yeah, and that was for my own safety and me own protection, but, um, in, in those days, in the, in 1969 to 73, uh, period, I was, um, I was a pretty mixed up kid. Um, I had a lot of things happen to me that I didn't like, and, um, I, um, [pause] yeah. I thought a bit different because of that, um, and because I wondered, you know, you don't, you don't seem to hear many stories about other people or other situations, you don't hear much on the news, you might hear, oh, the woman has been, um, abused by her partner or whatever, that might be the only thing that you hear, um, yeah, you don't hear, you don't hear things like sexual assault, um, unless there's a rape somewhere, or, uh, there's a paedophile on the loose, even then you might not hear it. Um, but, well yeah, if you put two and two together come up with an answer, your answer might be the person could be guilty, may be guilty of another sex, uh, crime against a young child because they've been interviewed, and the police know that that person is a paedophile. Uh, but you should never, ever assume, uh, that's the case because they may be innocent. Just because they're a paedophile doesn't mean they're gonna, uh, go out and, well, that person might not be the person that's done it. You know, there may be somebody else, I don't know. [pause] I don't know what a paedophile's life's like, and I don't want to know. As far as I'm concerned you should chop their dicks off, then they can't do anything.

Here Roger is in an unstable position in relation to what he is trying to describe and whether he wants to tell me about the event or not. As he mentions—'you don't seem to hear many stories about other people or other situations'— Roger did not have access to a discourse, because it is invisible. Perhaps it is an abjected experience or position that he is unable to verbalise. If abjection is a social practice impressed on the bodies of individuals, perhaps those individuals come to feel responsible for their own abjection, and they are consequently too ashamed to recount it. When Roger also talks about abjecting others—chopping the dicks off paedophiles—his anger and violence emerge again. It is also interesting that he conceived the people he needed to be protected from in prison were his 'friends'. This trope of misplaced friendship occurs in other narratives collected in this research (Amal, Jake, and Peter), and is echoed in the wider literature (see Landman 2014; Thomas 2011). Given the institutional contexts in which Roger, Amal, Jake, and Peter have built their friendships,[7] friendship is also an experience of abjection. They are at permanent threat of abjection—even from 'friends'—which exposes the precarity of their lives.

My memory, my field notes, and the next question I asked all indicate that Roger's unexplained and somewhat opaque account confused me. I responded as best I could:

(So I'm a little bit lost, so what are we talking about?)

Um, I'm not sure what I'm talking about now, I'm just mumbling. Um, [pause] I think I was, I think I was trying to answer your question in a roundabout way. Um, when I said that, um, I don't like, uh, things that have happened to me in the past, whether it be in the institution or no matter where it is. Um, when I found out, uh, something in my file from the boys' home, um, what happens, in, in, uh, what happens in the gaols, and what happens with paedophiles, and what paedophiles do. Um, uh, [pause] so long as it doesn't go any further, I was raped. I could not prove that I wasn't raped. That's how I ended up in gaol, but that's not to go any further than this room.[8]

It is interesting how Roger broached the topic in a 'roundabout way', as if he did not want to answer explicitly nor go into much detail (or because he did not have the language to articulate it in the way he desired). His uncertainty is understandable because, like Deb, perhaps if he discloses his experience of rape, it compounds his feelings of abjection. Simultaneously, he knows what happened to him in the past when he told someone—he was not believed and in some ways was held responsible and incarcerated. Maybe he feels cheated and unsure. *Will Ryan believe me? What will Ryan think of me? What will Ryan do?*

Roger also framed these events as 'things he didn't like', perhaps minimising the real harm caused, or to preserve his own well-being. In the second interview, Roger also made a reference to an event at the boys' home, but this was not explored further. At the time I thought it was inappropriate to go into too much detail about the incident, so I waited until our fourth interview. I appreciated the fact that Roger had disclosed small pieces of information throughout each interview, perhaps not wanting to dwell on it too much because it was still deeply traumatic for him. He may have also wanted to test me and my reactions; after all, we learned previously how he was wary of people when he first met them. Roger's crip time works through disclosure and excision; he discloses and forecloses information over time.

I came to learn in our fourth interview that a man aged somewhere around 50 years old, and a frequenter of the 'drunks' refuge, raped Roger in a toilet block. Roger did not know the man, except he had seen him around before. Roger was asked if he went to the police:

No I was too scared. I didn't even know it was a crime. Somehow the police found out, I don't know how, uh, and they came to the [refuge] and started asking me questions and then took me to the police station. They got me to make a statement, you know, I was talking about what I thought, or, you know, this happened, that happened, the police put words, it's like they were putting words in me mouth. But, I don't know if they were or not, but, yeah. And then they, uh, asked me to sign it.

Roger did not go to the police because he was in a state of abject fear, and because he did not know it was a crime (corresponding with Deb's experiences). 'Homosexuality'[9] was illegal in the state of Victoria until 1980, and Roger's rape occurred around 1969. That Roger did not know he was a victim of a crime is indicative of spending most of his life in an asylum; he is unaware of some social norms and legal rules that are more pervasively understood in public discourse (to an extent at least, recognising this was in the 1960s). The police have also compounded his abjection by manipulating him into admitting he engaged in consensual 'homosexual' sex.

He was asked what he thought the offender's motivations were for this form of heterotopic violence:[10]

I think he thought I was vulnerable. I think he thought that, um, you know, there's something not quite right about this person. Um, I think he also thought because he shouted me food and whatnot that I owed it to him, you know, so yeah.

Roger understands that other people think he is different. Like Deb, Roger also speculates that the violence is a transaction for a deed they have provided. Disabled people are so abjected that some abled people merely use them to get whatever benefit they want (see Sherry 2010; Thomas 2011). On another occasion, Roger said,

Well, I'm sure it was because of my disability. Because that person saw that I could be, you know, a bit slow with something, I don't know. There's something different about me.

Roger points to the incompatibility between his crip time and standard time, suggesting he is 'slow' intellectually. Notwithstanding the fact that all people go through changes concerning intellectual development throughout their lives, these differences are taken to only apply, and to matter, to disabled people (Titchkosky 2007). Roger also suggests there is something 'different' about him, and while *difference* may certainly be embraced (claiming *crip* may be one such example), in this exchange, it appeared to me that he was talking about difference in a negative and reductive sense. Given the ways in which the agents in the asylums have continually told Roger he is not normal, and that this abnormality is negative, it is possible to see how Roger comes to view himself as negatively deviating from the norm, and he perceives he is treated 'not-normally'.

It was obvious that these processes of abjection were deeply traumatic for Roger to re-live. He was asked how he healed from the incident:

> Um, I don't really because I haven't really had counselling around, around this, um. I think I keep pushing it back and back and back into the back of my brain, you know. And then back into the subconscious kind of area, whatever that is. Um, I'd often thought about whether, whether I should get counselling or not about it, but then it's almost like you feel dirty, and, you know, it's almost like you're, I don't know what the word is, I keep seeing the vision of me in that toilet block, um. I asked him not to, um, I didn't want to, um, but he just kept on going and almost, it's almost like he was forcing himself, um, that's what made me say to the police that I didn't, I told him I didn't want to, I didn't want to, I didn't want to, and it was like he was forcing himself on me. 'Oh no you didn't, you know, you're a willing party, you're, you're part of the crime, you're, you're just as dirty and filthy as he is'. Um, so hence I was charged, to this day I still don't know why, but never mind.

In Roger's account, not only did the offender force himself onto Roger, but the police forced Roger into admitting guilt, which compounded his abjection. Roger's imperative is to think little about this ordeal—cast it from memory—and try to forget about it, move on with life, and 'never mind'.

His reference to feeling 'dirty' is illuminating and aligns with Douglas (1966: 36) aphorism that dirt is 'matter out of place'. According to Douglas (1966), dirt is defined as that which is morally impure according to specific spatial and temporal factors. Douglas (1966: 2) writes that dirt 'offends against order'. Dirt is something that is not absolute; rather, dirt 'confuse[s] or contradict[s] cherished classifications' (Douglas 1966: 37). She writes,

> [s]hoes are not dirty in themselves, but it is dirty to place them on the dining-table, food is not dirty in itself, but it is dirty to leave cooking utensils in the bedroom, or food bespattered on clothing; similarly, bathroom equipment in the drawing room; clothing lying on chairs; out-door things in-doors; upstairs things downstairs; under-clothing appearing where over-clothing should be, and so on.
>
> (Douglas 1966: 37)

Within this context, not only is Roger out of place in society (because of his disabled subjectivity), he also feels dirty because he is involved in an act— male/male rape—that is doubly out of place amongst social norms. Various dimensions of abjection have compounded and pressed upon him; he is disabled, raped by a man, and presumed gay. For Roger, 'feeling dirty' may be an effort to abjectify himself in order to preserve his own subjectivity. That is, Roger must cast out that which he finds repulsive in order to re-establish his sense of bodily integrity. In this sense, Roger has experienced abjection, but also abjectifies/expunges the remnants of 'homosexuality' and 'homosexual sex' lingering from the encounter, and from which it remains 'dirty'.

When Roger was asked how the incident came to the attention of the police, he speculated that someone had seen them in the toilet block or the man had told the police himself. After all, this man was apparently in trouble with the law for several other incidents. Sensing that we had reached a point where Roger had told me all he wanted about the incident, we moved to another topic. At the end of our fourth interview, Roger asked me not to ask him any more questions about this event in our last interview. His wishes were obviously respected, and I appreciated his candour nevertheless. Rather than 'cast it off' and abjectify himself or the event, Roger kept it inside him at a distance. In this sense, his memories of the event occupy an abject space in his mind that he separates from himself.

As stipulated by the judge's order, after a month in prison, Roger checked into another asylum. He stayed there for about five months, and it is clear that Roger did not cope well:

> I used to play up in there, and knock my hands around, cut me wrists, and Christ knows what, run away a couple of times, and, yeah.

These violent actions of self-harm are explicit examples of self-abjection: trying to cast out that which he perceives intolerable. Roger's description that he is 'play[ing] up' also points to ways in which his self-abjection has been normalised and minimised. He is embodying social attitudes about his disabled subjectivity—that have worked their way through all of the institutions Roger has occupied—and he is abjecting himself because he is outcast.

While Roger was initially a voluntary patient, he was eventually certified. Again, how this happened remains unclear. The asylum was only designed for temporary stays, so Roger was moved to another institution where he lived for somewhere around five years. Upon his eventual release, Roger was again struggling emotionally:

> when I came out, I found it really hard…I was fairly, really suicidal, I was hearing voices, or what I thought was hearing voices. Um, I didn't know anybody. I was alone in the world. Um, had no money to go see me mother. So I sat on the, on the, on the bridge…I sat on the, on the bridge there with my legs dangling over. The police came and, and pulled me off, told me off and, they, they, they find out I had medication in my pocket. I was gonna take some just before I jumped. So, and it had the hospital's name on, so they presumed I'd, I'd come from there. So they ended up taking me back there again.

Roger was in a state of abjection, hearing voices, self-harming, and suicidal. He was alone in the world and saw little option but to commit suicide. These thoughts of suicide also entered *Peter Camilleri's* narrative, who was bullied relentlessly by 'friends' and family. *Clifton Murphy* contemplated suicide too, after years of bullying from his family and strangers. Ultimately, the disabled asylums worsened Roger's emotional state. As the purpose of these asylums is to regulate people to achieve normalcy, and because Roger knows and is told that he can never be normal, suicide and depression become more of a possibility than normality.

Roger's predicament also raises several important implications for the relationship between suicide and abjection. If, in a Kristevan (1982) sense, the corpse is the ultimate site of the abject ('the utmost of abjection' [Kristeva 1982: 4]), then suicide itself surely sits as one of the ultimate acts of abjection—expunging the self from the social organism completely and permanently. Whereas abjection typically involves 'casting off' to preserve bodily integrity, the process of suicide is about casting off to *destroy* integrity. While Kristeva (1982: 2) suggests that the abject 'does not cease challenging its master', one exception to this rule appears to be suicide. Abjection is the 'friend that stabs you' (Kristeva 1982: 4), and in the moment of suicide, the precariousness of bodies is exposed; like abjection, we see the collapse of self and body, nature and culture, life and death (Kristeva 1982).

Roger's stories were so characterised by (involuntary) movement between asylums that it was difficult to trace what types of experiences he had in these zones (other than those at the training farm). When I put this question to him, he related a few experiences. Unfortunately, I am not able to determine where or when they happened, and Roger may not even know himself. I do not know how many asylums Roger occupied throughout his life. Given Roger left the room adjacent to the boys' home at 19 years of age and was finally de-institutionalised somewhere around his twenty-third birthday, these events happened roughly somewhere between 1967 and 1973. The stories expose his (stolen and) cripped time; they are told in a fragmented and chaotic fashion. Contrasting Deb's stories, these stories show how Roger struggled to navigate, and make sense of, institutional life. This is not to say that Deb did not struggle over making sense of her experiences, but rather that she recounted her history in a way that drew connections between people, events, motives, practices, and feelings. For Roger, on the other hand, the fragments of his life history never quite seemed to add up, such that they made little sense to him. This senselessness both constitutes and intensifies his abjection. He described a moment of institutional life thus:

> one particular day, I was in love with this girl, um, [Jennifer]. And we liked each other. And I got told off by the, one of the staff for, not going back to what I'm supposed to be going back to. And I was. I was on my way back to the kitchen, because I was on kitchen duty. Which he might know, if he'd a looked at the roster on the, on the boards, he woulda known. Anyway, I turned round and started yelling and screaming at him, and next thing I remember, I'm waking up

laying on the bed with this dirty big hang-, dirty big hangover, and headache, and my head was sore. And the reason my head was sore was that I'd cut my head open, because I'd run smack bang into the wall. 'Cause as I yelled at him, he turned, wanted to know what, what was going on, and because he had moved, and because I was running so fast, I didn't have time to stop so, of course I knocked myself out, which I didn't know until I'd been told later. I had scans done, ECGs and whatnot, they'd put me on Tegretol thinking that I was an epileptic, but that didn't prove anything. They had me on all these medications, zonking me out, and I didn't like that.

What made him get angry? Why did they think he had epilepsy? Roger's life history narrative is frequently shaped by experiences of anger and violence. It has been difficult to trace his movements—and the reasons for them. In this anecdote, it is difficult again to get any sense of context. Perhaps the medications throughout his institutionalisation have *cripped* his time, leaving him hazy on details and explanations? Perhaps he is ashamed of his conduct and does not want to tell me. Perhaps Roger does not know himself.

Roger told me another story from his time in the asylums:

I remember one incident though was that I was laying on the grass and, I was waiting for my lady friend to come, and, eventually she came and we sat on the grass together and we're just talking…Two nurses came, grabbed hold of me, took me to the [ward], and give me a needle, and that was the end of that. Until the next morning. I seen the doctor the next morning, he said 'geez you've been a bad boy'. Until this very day, I still don't know what I've supposed to have done. All the answers that I got was 'you know what you're done, you've been very, very naughty'. That's all the answers that I got. Maybe mistaken identity, I don't know.

Agents of abjection have knocked Roger out. *Why? How?* We do not know. They have also infantilised him—he is a 'bad boy'.[11] Roger later told me he had shock 'treatment' in the asylums and 'pills shoved down our throats', so it may be that his storytelling is fragmented and chaotic because he cannot remember with clarity what happened to him.[12] In trying to regulate Roger, the agents of abjection intensified his abjection and compromised his humanity and agency. *Where does this leave the abject body? How does he, and how can he, make sense of his life?*

When Roger was finally de-institutionalised around 1973, he went to visit his mother who worked at an accommodation service for elderly people. Roger was allowed to stay in a room of a converted barn. Again, he is in a zone that is outside the norm, one in which he never quite fits. At this point, Roger's life entered a degree of greater stability. Perhaps after years of institutional life Roger finally found some freedom and a place to call home. Roger started going to a Christian-run kitchen, purchasing food, drinking coffee, eating biscuits, playing cards, and talking with others almost every night of the week. Perhaps Roger had become habituated to the regimentation endemic to institutional life, and this institutionalised behaviour is another technology through which he copes with the 'outside world'. Eventually Roger met a girl, and they started going out together. They moved in with each other and became engaged. One night, however, after Roger visited his ill mum, he got home to find a note saying he needed to move out. Just when he thinks things are stable, his life, again, is dynamic.

Roger often described his mum with ambivalence, and in our third interview I asked him about his relationship with her:

> Oh my mum, um, I, I, I'm ashamed to say this and, and she's now passed away and I unfortunately couldn't get to talk to her about it, but, um, I'd often talk to her about my dad and, um, she always used to tell me that my dad had died in a motorbike accident, on the way to see her in hospital. She was having me, and he got word, um, because he was out on a boat doing something, I don't know what he was doing, fishing or whatever, and he came back, got on his motorbike to go to the hospital to see mum and, um, he got killed on the motorbike on the way to the, to see me mum. That's what she kept telling me. And then, uh, one day she was telling me that, um, the person in the photo is not my real dad. I'm saying 'what? [pause] You married him he's gotta be me real dad'. She said 'no he's not', she said 'what happened was that while I was still married with your dad, I actually had an affair', and she ended up getting pregnant to that, to that person. So that person is my father, not the one in the picture. And when the, my, the dad in the picture found out, he divorced me mother. Now in those days, it's a shame to bring shame on your family and your parents, to find out your mother, uh, who has got a child without a father. Um, and I think the word is you'd call, is that you're a bastard. Now I absolutely hate that word, hate it with a passion... Um, so, ever since, ever since then I've felt like me mother wasn't me mother. And, she's just someone who was looking after me, because, I don't know, maybe, maybe my real mother couldn't look after me, maybe she give it up, give, give me up. I, I, I don't know the reasons why, you know, so, my mother and I had a very, very rocky relationship.

It is unclear when Roger learned the truth about his father, but it is clear he felt betrayed. It is also another example of his world being turned upside down, time (with his father) stolen from him, and truth denied. Perhaps Roger's account of the truth of his life is so chaotic, fragmented, and shifting because his own truths, and those told to him, are also constantly changing. Just when something seems stable, his world starts shifting.

It was difficult to get a firm sense from Roger what he has done with his life after de-institutionalisation post-1973. He often spoke in generalities rather than specifics. I did learn that he was married then divorced, moved interstate then back again, and struggled to deal with his mum's ill health and death. Roger did not seem much interested in discussing these topics. When asked about his life since the mid-1970s, he spoke more about his emotions than actual events. When asked about things he had to overcome in life, he reflected on leaving the asylum for the final time:

> Um, probably getting out of the institution was the biggest one, because I was absolutely, I wanted to get out, but I was absolutely scared of what was out there, and, and the fear of people knowing that I've, I've come from an institution or I looked different, sounded different, talk different, perhaps some medication that I'm taking, um, that really petrified me and that really scared me.

Roger was simultaneously scared of the asylums and the outside world. He is in a predicament: the asylum is normal for him, yet he knows it is also a harmful place and not a normal zone for most (normal) people. He is also worried that he looks marked, whether through 'look', 'sound', or 'talk', and that people may know that he came from an asylum. This is also echoed in Deb's narrative, where both are scared that the locations they came from might be physically and visibly inscribed on the body.

Roger also said later,

> in the institution and in the boys' home, you didn't have to worry about a single thing. Everything was done for you, that is my safety net, that's my blanket, you know, my safety blanket.

This echoes Kristeva's (1982: 137) description that the abject is 'a security blanket'; for Roger, he knows he has always been abject, and his institution-alisation has become so normalised that he depends on it for his own abjection. Notwithstanding the harms the asylum brought Roger, the asylum has protected him from the uncertainty of the outside world. While Roger is abject in the asylum, he is used to that particular form of abjection, and does not have to imagine how the outside world would perceive his abject subject position. I asked him about the idea that some people may know about his time in the asylum, and he said,

> That's how I felt. That was probably just paranoia, what's called para-noia or whatever that bloody word is, you know, it was part of my inse-curity, I suppose, mate.

Disabled people are ubiquitously marked, defined, and inscribed through social practice as deficient and different, such that Roger has a fear that his 'difference' follows him around and may perhaps even be a corporeal mark. Roger's rejection of psy-disciplines is also evidenced here; whenever he mentions anything related to psychology or psychiatry, he gets angry: 'paranoia' is a 'bloody word', he had to see 'bloody psychs', and psychologists/ psychiatrists come from the 'nut factory'. Roger understands that psy-disciplines have pathologised him.

I mentioned earlier that Roger spoke about emotions rather than events when he reflected on his life post-1973. Roger told me that he often talks to others, including researchers, about his life in disabled asylums. It may be the case that he has rehearsed these stories so much that it is unexpected when he is asked about other parts of his life, and he does not have the 'script' to talk about these things. The shock 'treatment' may have also inhibited his memory, or maybe he simply did not want to talk about such things. In any event, here I foreground a couple of quotes that illuminate the emotions of which Roger spoke. When asked about any mistakes he made throughout his life, he replied:

> Um, being angry with the whole world and the whole system, and I wanna challenge the whole world and the whole system, and to say, you know 'Fuck this!' You know, excuse the expression, but it, it, some of it is wrong. Some of it is wrong with the way that people with disability are treated. Some of it is wrong with the way of, that normal society, whatever 'normal' is, is treated. Why is it that we can't be treated the same as any other normal person in this community? Why can't we have the same basic human rights?

Roger is obviously very passionate about the rights of disabled people. He is angry that disabled people are treated unequally, and the stories he told me are certainly evidence of this. I was unclear why he spoke about his maltreatment when I had asked him about mistakes he had made in his life. Perhaps he thinks it is a mistake the way that society treats disabled people, or maybe he thinks his life has been one big mistake. Or perhaps he simply wanted to answer a different question (see Scheurich 1995) and did not want to reflect on his own mistakes.

Roger accepts he is not normal, yet nevertheless desires to be treated normally. On another occasion he said,

> Can you really wonder why I get angry when, when things that, you know, when we have to fight for things? You know that, the, the advocacy movement, you know we're having to fight for our, for what we want, you know.

Roger's main passion now is his advocacy work. After years of violence, Roger is trying to redirect his anger to advocacy work, trying to turn bad into good (reminiscent of Deb's 'good/winning' side not 'bad/losing' side).

Having spent time in more than six asylums in his earlier life, it is clear that Roger likes the simple things now. At the time of our last interview, Roger told me he enjoys his self-advocacy work and his relationship with Lisa. Thirteen months after our last interview, however, I learned that his relationship with Lisa has ended; more movement, more change. He also told me he likes watching television (old shows, particularly). After all the turbulent years, I asked Roger if he felt like he was finally in control of his life:

> Do I feel I'm in control of my life? No. Because if I felt like I was in control of my life, then I don't think I'd be having any anger issues. I don't think I'd be having, get frustrated and angry and really yelling and screaming, carrying on like a two-bob watch because of something I'm unhappy about.

Anger is still a part of *being Roger*, and it is also a form of his resistance. Roger also spends a lot of time thinking back on his life; I think trying to make sense of it. He wants to turn his life into a book. Perhaps reading back on things might help him connect some dots. He also enjoyed telling his story:

> I'm still angry and whatnot, but every time I'm telling my story, it's getting less and less and less. So it's like this big huge boulder that's been lifted off my shoulder and that, that's gone…I don't think I'm already pain-free because I've still got the memories, I know what it is like, you know. I can say to you that institutions are a rotten place, you were abused, you were raped, whatever, whatever, oh, 'surely that can't have happened'. But that's, that's my [emphasis] story, that's what happened when I was there. It may not be happening now, it may not happen in the future but that's what it did happen.

I cannot help but think of two things: the chaos in Roger's life, and all those people who cautioned that my research would be too traumatic for the participants. Roger wants to tell his story; he wants to heal and make sense of his life. He wants to turn around his injustices and show people who hear his stories what he experienced and what he got through. In this sense, Roger is now focussed on resistance: trying to reclaim his abjection, tell people what happened, and throw it back at society.

Considering Roger's story

What are we to make of Roger's life and story? While Deb has broken free from her abjection, for Roger this is not so clear. He has entered similar abjected zones to Deb, yet Roger's experiences are more chaotic and fractured. His abjection has been compounded, and his body regulated and violated. This exposes the multiplicity of abjection across shifting spatial and temporal contexts. Yet this does not mean there is no opportunity for Roger to reject/resist his abjection. For example, Deb broke free from her abjection by embracing her indigeneity (paradoxically, another socially abjected group). This gave Deb the ability to, in some ways, embrace abjection, to disarm it. *What might Roger be able to do?*

Before finding the self-advocacy movement in later life, Roger's strategy to resist abjection was his anger. At various times he fought back, ran away, refused to do tests, and hit out at others. Speculatively, perhaps he was using his anger as a strategy to move elsewhere, even if it was another institution. If he did not like where he was, he could fight against the system until they could not bear it. In this respect, for Roger, anger is resistance.

Today Roger is involved in the self-advocacy movement, and this might be Roger's way of resisting his, and other people's, abjection. It seems that Roger's life has entered a state of greater stability. He goes to his self-advocacy group throughout the week, has a few friends, and likes to live the 'simple life' watching TV on the couch. In fact, self-advocacy might be Roger's way of resisting his abjection. In a world where his rights have been stripped away and he has been dehumanised and abjected, self-advocacy becomes a space for Roger to reaffirm his humanness and vent his anger in a normalised way that helps him fight against injustice.

In both this and the previous chapter, I have focussed mostly on social abjection—that which is inflicted from others and on to disabled bodies. Informed by McClintock's (1995) framework, I have also analysed how multiple dimensions work to regulate and violate Roger in different temporal and spatial moments. While at this stage I have focussed on Deb and Roger, in the forthcoming chapter I introduce the reader to eleven new participants. I argue most of these new participants abjected themselves through pathologising and disavowing their disabled subjectivity. I consider these stories of self-abjection to demonstrate how ableist and disablist discourses work to regulate disabled subjects through the internalisation of negative assumptions about disabled embodiment. In so doing, I foreground a constitutive relation between the social and the psychic, the collective and the individual, in the production of an abject subject.

Notes

1 Throughout the course of this text, Davis (2013: 1, italics in original) departs from this claim and argues that '*diversity* is the new *normality*'.
2 A boys' home is commonly referred to as a boarding school in UK and US contexts.
3 Discussed later.
4 It is unclear what functions and purpose the training farm had. During this period of time, many training farms in Australia housed Aboriginal, migrant, and intellectually disabled children, and most training farms offered industrial schooling and farm training.
5 In comparing disabled people to docile bodies, I think it is important to qualify that I do not intend, and nor does Foucault, to suggest that docile bodies lack

agency. As Foucault (1977) affirms, while power and discourse work to regulate the body, humans possess ethical and moral dimensions to conform, or more importantly, resist, such norms. As Mansfield (2000: 63) writes, that as 'power/ knowledge works at the level of the subject, then it is at the level of the subject that it will most effectively be resisted'.

6 For some participants I introduced red and yellow signs; the red sign said 'Stop Interview', while the yellow sign said 'Next Question'. They were invited to hold up whichever sign whenever they desired.

7 Roger in the asylums, Amal and Jake at school, and Peter through extended family and friends.

8 After I had a conversation again with Roger about confidentiality and anonymity, he agreed that this story could be used in this book.

9 I am reluctant to use the word 'homosexual' or 'homosexuality'. It is a term that began to emerge within a medical and psychological discourse in the late nineteenth century (Foucault 1978). It is a term given to diagnose and define their/my/our difference. I find it an offensive and oppressive term, and consequently prefer the term 'gay man' or 'queer'. I am also reluctant because Roger did not define the experience in this way.

10 This refers, in a broad sense, to violence that occurs outside of everyday social and institutional spaces (Foucault 1986).

11 This also constitutes a form of adultism, which refers to the belief that adults are superior to children, and that children can be infantilised and regulated (Slater 2013, 2015; Stafford 2017).

12 Upon learning of Roger's shock 'treatment', I borrowed a medical book on 'electroconvulsive therapy' from the library (Abrams 1997). I read that the therapy (and 'therapy' is certainly a curious way to describe it) can lead to confusion, delirium, negative effects on memory, and so on (Abrams 1997).

References

Abrams, R 1997, *Electroconvulsive Therapy*, 3rd edition, Oxford University Press, New York and Oxford.

Davis, LJ 2013, *The End of Normal: Identity in a Biocultural Era*, The University of Michigan Press, Ann Arbor, MI.

Douglas, M 1966, *Purity and Danger: An Analysis of Concepts of Pollution and Taboo*, Routledge & Kegan Paul, London.

Foucault, M 1977, *Discipline and Punish: The Birth of the Prison*, Vintage Books, New York.

Foucault, M 1978, *The History of Sexuality, Vol. I: An Introduction*, translated by Robert Hurley, Pantheon Books, New York.

Foucault, M 1986, 'Of Other Spaces', *Diacritics*, 16(1): 22–27, translated by J Miskowiec.

Kristeva, J 1982, *Powers of Horror: An Essay on Abjection*, translated by LS Roudiez, Columbia University Press, New York.

Landman, RA 2014, '"A Counterfeit Friendship": Mate Crime and People with Learning Disabilities', *The Journal of Adult Protection*, 16(4): 355–366.

Mansfield, N 2000, *Subjectivity: Theories of the Self from Freud to Haraway*, Allen & Unwin, Sydney.

McClintock, A 1995, *Imperial Leather: Race, Gender and Sexuality in the Colonial Contest*, Routledge, New York and London.

Plummer, K 2001, *Documents of Life 2: An Invitation to Critical Humanism*, SAGE, London.

Scheurich, JJ 1995, 'A Postmodernist Critique of Research Interviewing', *International Journal of Qualitative Studies in Education*, 8(3): 239–252.

Sherry, M 2010, *Disability Hate Crimes: Does Anyone Really Hate Disabled People?*, Ashgate Publishing, Farnham, Surrey.

Slater, J 2013, 'Playing Grown-Up: Using Critical Disability Perspectives to Rethink Youth', in *Youth: Responding to Lives: An International Reader*, edited by A Azzopardi Sense Publishers, Rotterdam, pp. 75–91.

Stafford, L 2017, '"What about My Voice?" Emancipating the Voices of Children with Disabilities through Participant-Centred Methods', *Children's Geographies*, 15(5): 600–613.

Thomas, P 2011, '"Mate Crime": Ridicule, Hostility and Targeted Attacks against Disabled People', *Disability & Society*, 26(1): 107–111.

Titchkosky, T 2007, *Reading and Writing Disability Differently: The Textured Life of Embodiment*, University of Toronto Press, Toronto.

Warner, M 1999, *The Trouble with Normal: Sex, Politics, and the Ethics of Queer Life*, Harvard University Press, Cambridge, MA.

5   Eleven lives

In the preceding chapters, I have demonstrated some of the ways in which disablist and ableist violence can be reimagined as abjection by drawing on the life histories of Deb and Roger. To remind the reader, disablist violence re-instantiates negative assumptions of disability and disabled people, while ableist violence works to (re)produce the abled subject as the norm (Campbell 2009). I am theorising the ways in which practices of abjection constitute and regulate subjects psychically and socially, and how this abjection might be resisted. Thus far I have introduced the narratives of Deb and Roger, and in reflecting on their life histories, I have primarily focussed on abjection as a social practice. In Chapter 6, however, I interrogate the psychic dimension of abjection through engagement with the narrative life histories of ten participants. This chapter, then, re-introduces the people who participated in this research. In keeping with life history narrative research, I want to give a fuller account of the participants as living, breathing people. Omitting Deb and Roger (who you 'know' by now), I present some brief biographies of the remaining participants in the order in which I met them.

The process of crafting these stories took a great deal of reflection and contemplation. I was guided by Plummer's (2001) point that the purpose behind the writing should be considered before any text is written. My purpose was/is to inform the reader about the participant's lives, foreground what they chose to tell me, and to theorise violence as abjection. In reality, I wrote each narrative several times throughout the evolution of this project. It was not until I was confident that I accurately conveyed their authorial voice that I was satisfied with my narration.

Lisa Austin

Lisa Austin is a 34-year-old mother of one. She was born in Melbourne, and both of her parents are labelled intellectually and physically disabled. At 6 months of age Lisa was taken away from her parents and placed in the care of her grandmother, because, in Lisa's account, she was not fed properly. When Lisa was nine-and-a-half years old, she went back to her parents when her grandmother became ill. Her grandmother died soon after, and her mother became abusive towards Lisa. Lisa described the abuse as including physical, emotional, and psychological harm. Eventually, at 14 years of age, Lisa and her dad found alternative housing together. In addition to the abuse from her mother, Lisa was also bullied at school. For the first three years of schooling, Lisa went to a 'normal' school, then to a 'special' school thereafter. Lisa said she was bullied at both schools, yet the emphasis of the bullying was different. At the 'special' school, Lisa was bullied because she struggled to socialise with the other children, yet in the 'normal' school, she was bullied because she was a poor learner, or incapable of doing some things the other students could.

After high school Lisa went to live in a residential service. There she met a man, and it developed into a close friendship. They have a daughter together —Stephanie[1]—who, at the time of our interviews (May–September 2015), was 6 years old. The pregnancy was not planned, and Lisa said many people thought that she should not, or could not, have children. Many people were shocked when they found out she was pregnant. Lisa told me that Stephanie lives with her paternal grandmother, because a court ruled that Lisa and her (then) partner were incapable of raising a child. Child Protection Services told Lisa that she may unintentionally harm Stephanie, and Lisa fears that she may reproduce the abuse she experienced as a child. Lisa is only allowed to spend two hours per week with Stephanie, and this upsets her. Lisa and Stephanie's father have since separated. Today, Lisa is the President of a self-advocacy group for people labelled intellectually disabled, and she fights for the rights of disabled people, particularly parents. This role keeps her busy, so when she has free time, she enjoys playing computer games and relaxing with her partner, Roger.[2]

Jake Hawkins

Jake Hawkins is a 22-year-old Sydney man, and most of what we spoke about revolved around school and bullying. As we only spoke once, details are limited. Jake said he had plenty of friends growing up, until Facebook entered the frame. On Facebook, he was bullied by other students he thought were his 'friends'. In Jake's account, schoolchildren would message him on Facebook and call him terms such as 'useless', 'idiot', and 'stupid'. The online bullying moved into the school arena where they would verbally bully him and throw things like sticks at him. He told teachers and his parents, but he was commonly told to simply ignore them. Jake's emotions varied, where he wanted to 'kill' or 'bash' his bullies, run away, or ignore them. At one stage he moved to another school in response to the bullying. Another time one of his bullies was suspended. The bullying stopped when Jake left high school, and three years after deleting his Facebook account, he now has a new one. He is more diligent about whom he befriends, and if anyone causes trouble, he just blocks them.

Jake does work placements through a disability employment provider, and he has his learner's license and a girlfriend. He still lives at home with his mum and dad, and Jake's older sister has moved out of home. He has a good relationship with his parents, and he enjoys playing ten-pin bowling with them for fun. Jake thinks that society does not fairly treat disabled people, and he thinks this is wrong. After one interview Jake chose to take no further part in this research. My feeling was that he had said all he had wanted to say and did not think he needed to elaborate any further.

Anne-Marie Holloway

In the second last chapter, I introduce *Anne-Marie Holloway's* life history, so in this section, I keep her biographical details brief. Anne-Marie is 43 years old, and she lives in Sydney. Throughout our interviews together, Anne-Marie focussed her story on two things: her experiences of domestic violence, and the violence and bullying she received from the police when reporting that violence. In her private life, Anne-Marie enjoys spending time with her dad, going to the beach, horse riding, sewing, collecting antique clocks, music, eating pasta, making cakes, and catching up with friends for coffee.

Amal Alam

Amal Alam is 35 years old and was born and resides in Sydney. She is Lebanese-Australian and belongs to a family of nine children, mum, and dad (two siblings passed away at early ages). Amal is blind, as are two other sisters. When Amal was younger, her family travelled both nationally and internationally looking for cures, yet they have been told it is incurable because it is a genetic condition. Despite this, Amal often experiences strangers walking up to her to tell her otherwise. These people tell Amal that 'they' (read professionals/doctors) will find a cure for her in a few years, ask her personal questions such as the cause of her blindness, and inquire whether she will ever have a family. Amal finds these questions acceptable or otherwise depending on the context and nature of the questions. She is frustrated, however, that people ignore her when she is shopping, and people constantly ask her why she is walking around without a guide dog.

Amal was bullied throughout her schooling. She said this occurred because other students did not understand her, and she did not understand them. The other students would hide things from her, draw things on her, and tell her the wrong information. The bullying took quite a toll on Amal, and she received little support from the school or her parents. The most typical advice Amal received was the suggestion to simply ignore it.

After school, Amal left her 'friends' behind and sought employment prospects. Today she works five days a week, four at a sheltered workshop,[3] and one day volunteering at an organisation that assists people with blindness or low vision. Amal said it is easier trying to find work in supported employment rather than the open market.

During our conversations Amal spoke about daily interactions with the world, where she has been subjected to several instances of violence. This includes extreme forms such as an incident of stalking, and being verbally abused as a child because she and her two blind sisters could have caused an 'accident' in public. Amal has also engaged in online dating, yet men have abused her and asked her for money when they learn of her disability. Amal is no longer seeking a relationship.

Amal also enjoys travelling; she has been to Europe, Tasmania, and Melbourne. She and her family are currently saving to go on another holiday. Amal describes herself as a happy person, yet she is cautious about making new friends. She relies a lot on the support of her family.

Emma Silva

Emma Silva is a 32-year-old woman who was born in England. She is a sole child and has not seen her father since she was a baby. Emma moved to Sydney, Australia, with her mum when she was 6 months old. Emma says that she has a neurological disability (epilepsy), autism spectrum disorder, learning disability, and a psychiatric disability (anxiety). Emma says the doctors class her as 'dual diagnosis', meaning she needs various support for differing needs. Emma describes herself as stubborn, and she relishes routine, structure, and clarity. If anything planned for Emma is altered, her day is thrown off balance.

Throughout our four interviews, Emma focussed mostly on bureaucratic issues in her life: employment, education, and public transport. Emma has difficulty finding employment. When she does find a job, she says her employers give her inflexible working hours, tell her she does not know her place and constantly steps out of line, and say that she does work that is outside her area of responsibility. Emma is currently unemployed because she cannot find the right job for her.

Emma goes to TAFE (Technical and Further Education) to help develop her skills for finding employment. Again, Emma finds TAFE non-accommodating, as she is only supported for a limited number of hours per week, and she considers the support she does receive to be inadequate. She is also unhappy that she cannot select the support worker she wants. Emma also cited public transport as a big issue, where trains do not stop long enough to allow her to board safely and bus drivers are sometimes rude to her.

Emma told me that her mum died when she was eleven, and that she was then raised by her nan (grandmother). When her nan died in 2001, 16-year-old Emma went to live with her aunt and uncle, and she still lives with them today. Emma misses her mum and nan very much. Emma owns and drives a car but still relies on public transport a lot because parking can be difficult in certain locations. Emma has a few friends, and she likes to go to the movies with them, have lunch, or catch up for coffee. Emma is also involved in a self-advocacy group, and she comes into the office once a week to help oversee things. Emma has never been on a date, and she has no intention of being in a relationship. The happiest times of Emma's life were holiday trips to New Zealand in 2012 and England in 2013.

Freddie Watkins

Freddie Watkins is a tall, brooding, 50-year-old man who was born and lives in Sydney. He is brooding because everything around him seems to be going wrong, at least that is what he told me at our first and only interview. At the time of our interview in September 2015, Freddie had not seen his 8-year-old son for thirteen months. According to Freddie, he divorced his wife in 2012 following turbulence in the relationship, which included the rumour that she had been intimate with another man. Freddie says his wife will not let him see their son because the son has bad asthma, and she does not think he can take proper care of him. Freddie thinks this is just an excuse, and he is thinking about pursuing some legal options to try and see his son.

Freddie now lives on his own, and his neighbours do not talk to him, preferring instead to socialise amongst themselves. Freddie does not mind this, however, as he prefers to keep to himself. Freddie likes to either catch up with his own friends, go to the library to borrow movies, or go for walks. While Freddie's mum and dad have died, he does have three older brothers and a sister. He only speaks to two of them, as the others do not want anything to do with Freddie. Freddie does not know why this is the case.

When I sat down with Freddie for the second time, our interview did not eventuate. He said he was really 'cut up' about what we had previously spoken about and had kept thinking about it since. Freddie and I decided together that we would draw his participation in this research to a close.

Joshua Rodgers

Joshua Rodgers is 24 years old and was born in Sydney. He grew up surrounded by his mum, dad, and two older sisters. All members of the family, except one sister, are labelled 'intellectually disabled'. When Joshua was in primary school, his parents divorced, so he went to live with his dad and still resides with him. Joshua maintains a good relationship with his family, and his parents have a positive relationship.

Joshua focussed a lot of his story on childhood bullying at school. He has a lisp, and students would mock Joshua for the way he talked. They would get Joshua to read out passages over and over again because apparently the way Joshua talked was 'funny'. Joshua's nickname was 'Spedley', a pejorative term that was a portmanteau of 'special' and 'education'. Joshua was bullied emotionally and assaulted physically. The advice given to him by his parents and teachers was to ignore it. Joshua said he struggled to deal with the bullying, and it made him eat more and put on a lot of weight. He struggled to control his anger, and sometimes snapped at people, and head-butted and punched brick walls in moments of rage. As a result of counselling sessions and art therapy, Joshua can now better manage his anger.

Once year eleven came around, things were better for Joshua as most of the bullies had left school. After high school Josh enrolled in TAFE. He studied Hospitality (he loves cooking), English, Horticulture, and now he studies Disability. This has created a passion in Joshua, where he now wants to fight for disabled people and promote anti-bullying in schools. Joshua is the Vice President at a self-advocacy service for people labelled 'intellectually disabled'.

Joshua also identifies as bisexual, and this has caused some trouble and apprehension for him in the past. Some people have mistreated him when he told them, and so he used to be cautious about whom he told. These days, however, he feels things have changed, and he is open and honest about this. Joshua perceives that society is more accepting of non-heterosexual people than disabled people, and consequently, he is more worried about disclosing he is disabled than being bisexual.

Today Joshua still goes to TAFE, and he hopes to fight for the lives of disabled people through his self-advocacy work. He has had his learner driver's license for three years now, and he will soon go for his provisional license when he has more time to practice. Joshua enjoys socialising with his small family and friendship network.

Peter Camilleri

Peter Camilleri is a shy and reserved 57 year old who has spent his entire life in Sydney. He is Maltese-Australian, is the youngest of two children, and resides in his parents' home alone following both their deaths in 2015. During his childhood, Peter had health problems including asthma and constant chest infections. He went to a 'special' school, then a 'mainstream' school. He was bullied at the latter school and sometimes beaten up, and his parents and teachers told him to ignore it.

After high school, Peter got a job at a pool factory where he drove forklifts and made deliveries. Two years later they closed, so Peter got another job driving trucks. He has been doing this on and off ever since. A few years ago, he also set up a mowing business cutting people's lawns. He has about forty clients, but he is hoping this will increase.

During our interviews Peter disclosed that he had contemplated suicide because a few years ago, he was being bullied by his friends and family. In Peter's account, they bullied him about his appearance and intellectual disability, and they would do it to his face and behind his back at parties. He said most of them were either friends or cousins, and after he confronted them about it, he has chosen not to socialise with them anymore. Peter also told me a story where his brother tried to sell his house out from under him. Peter only found out when his solicitor rang to tell him. Since this emerged, Peter has had a strained relationship with his brother.

Peter likes spending time with his partner, Debbie,[4] who he has been with for about fifteen years. He says that he was a very shy person, but his involvement with self-advocacy has helped him open up a bit more. He likes going to the speedway with Debbie to watch car racing and going to the local club to have dinner, a drink, and a play on the pokies.

Warren Goodwin

I introduced the reader to *Warren Goodwin* in the 'Beginnings' chapter, where I used an encounter with him to contextualise McClintock's (1995) dimensions of abjection. Warren is 58 years old, and he has spent his whole life in Melbourne. When we met he seemed to only want to talk about two things: being gay and the sexual assault he experienced. About six years prior to our first interview (September 2015), Warren was sexually assaulted by a nurse in an accommodation service. In Warren's account, he rang the accommodation service after the event, and the police were called. He told the police what happened and the incident proceeded to court, yet the alleged offender was found not guilty. The alleged offender was not fired from his job, but to Warren's comfort, the man no longer works in the industry. Warren was upset that nothing had been done about the incident, and he formed the view that he was not believed. He attributes his victimisation more to being gay than being disabled.

Warren is also very proud of his sexuality. He 'came out' in 1990, and the happiest times of his life include going to the Sydney Gay and Lesbian Mardi Gras, and Gay Games. Yet he has still suffered discrimination; he has been refused entry into gay bars (because the establishment was not wheelchair-accessible), and some patrons have claimed he is not gay, simply because he is disabled. He also says that his mum struggled to come to terms with his sexuality, and he only has contact with two of his four siblings.

After two short interviews, Warren had said all he wanted to say about these two things and drew his participation to a close.

Richard Brady

Richard Brady is 60 years old and the father of three children (one of whom is *Joshua Rodgers*). He was born in Sydney in 1957 and is one of seven children. At three-and-a-half years of age, Richard was placed in an asylum because his family could not look after him. He moved to another asylum when he was 10 years old, and he was finally released at 15 years of age.

Richard experienced awful things at both asylums and consequently does not like to talk to people about it. He considers it as something that is behind him. Upon his exit from the asylums, Richard went to live with his dad and step-mom. Richard said it took a while for him to adjust to the outside world, and said that he was followed around by his brothers because they were fearful he might get hurt by someone. Richard was a target for violence because in addition to the label 'intellectual disability', he also has hydrocephalus, which means he has noticeable physical differences. Over the years, Richard has had surgery to separate his fingers, have his face re-structured, and an eye socket moved. In his youth he was bashed, and others launched invectives at him such as 'retard', 'four eyes', and 'handi-capped'. These days he mostly receives stares from people, and it depends on the situation whether he responds or not.

Richard devotes most of his time to self-advocacy work where he trains people how to engage with disabled people and promote their rights. Rich-ard married over two decades ago and has three children. When Richard and his wife were expecting their first child, Richard said many people told them they should not have children because it would be like 'a child having a child'. Richard likes proving people wrong, and he and his wife have suc-cessfully managed to raise their three children. While Richard is now divorced, the whole family still enjoy a positive relationship with each other.

According to Richard, he has not seen his biological mum for over ten years and is unsure if she is still alive. He also only communicates with one brother. He describes himself as stubborn and busy, and in addition to his work, he enjoys camping, ten-pin bowling, music, and movies. He is also very proud of his children.

Clifton Murphy

Clifton Murphy is 55 years of age and was born and lives in Sydney. In add-ition to the label 'intellectual disability', Clifton has right-sided cerebral palsy. In our interviews, he documented a deprived upbringing, where he was severely neglected by his parents. In Clifton's account, his parents thought he was a 'reject', and only provided him with food and no love. Clifton describes that everyone else in the family ate food from a plate, but he ate from a small saucer. Additionally, Clifton describes one incident where his mum tried to kill him.

Today, Clifton's parents are both dead, and he does not care, suggesting they should have loved him more. In response to his family's neglect, Clifton spent his childhood with animals and nature. He spent time with dogs, worms, ants, and birds, and he loved being outside. Clifton was also bashed and bul-lied at school. As far as Clifton is concerned, animals are better than people because animals do not hurt you. Clifton's passion for animals continued into adulthood. He has worked as an animal technician, and had jobs at pounds, zoos, and wildlife and national parks. Clifton has looked after many animals, including rats, mice, guinea pigs, rabbits, cats, dogs, sheep, horses, monkeys, orangutans, and more. He has not worked for over a decade now because of a workplace injury he received that affected his arm.

Clifton says he does not belong in society, where people think he is nothing, a joke, and a spastic. While Clifton has been married once, it ended in divorce after about twelve years. Clifton excludes himself from society because he thinks disabled people are not valued. He has also contemplated suicide. Clifton says he is open and honest and perceives life as a daily struggle. Clifton has become a Jehovah's Witness and spends his days with animals and nature. He wanted to tell me, and others, about his negative experiences because he thinks it is important to tell people what happens to disabled people and how they are treated.

Conclusion

I have offered these short biographies for two reasons: to give an account of these eleven people in a way that captures how they narrated their lives, and to offer their stories as a prologue to, and contextualisation of, the next chapter. In continuing my account of abjection, in the next chapter, I draw upon the excerpts of many of these participants to examine the interiority of abjection, framed through the ways in which they pathologised and disavowed their disabled subjectivities.

Notes

1 Not her real name.
2 As mentioned previously, Lisa and Roger have since separated.
3 This refers to an institution that only employs disabled people.
4 Not her real name.

References

Campbell, FK 2009, *Contours of Ableism: The Production of Disability and Ableness*, Palgrave Macmillan, London and New York.
McClintock, A 1995, *Imperial Leather: Race, Gender and Sexuality in the Colonial Contest*, Routledge, New York and London.
Plummer, K 2001, *Documents of Life 2: An Invitation to a Critical Humanism*, SAGE Publications, London.

6 (Psychic) Self-abjection
Pathologisation and disavowal

In Deb and Roger's chapters, I devoted my account of the abject to the ways in which exterior forces of abjection work on disabled bodies. By theorising violence as abjection, I have considered how tangible and explicit acts operate to violate and regulate disabled subjects. In this chapter, however, I consider how exterior forces of abjection work their way into the psychic life of disabled bodies. It is important that

> an account of subjection…must be traced in the turns of psychic life. More specifically, it must be traced in the peculiar turning of a subject against itself that takes place in acts of self-reproach, conscience, and melancholia that work in tandem with processes of social regulation.
>
> (Butler 1997a: 18–19)

Butler (1997a) suggests that social practices constitute one's psychic life, and in this chapter, I explore the simultaneous interrelation between the psychic and the social, the interior and the exterior, the singular and the collective. As Butler (2000) argues, social norms and practices are produced through a psychic enactment of the ideal, which is a fantasy simultaneously produced in un/conscious spheres. Just as Butler (1990, 1993) has documented how subjects are constituted through regulatory norms, in this chapter I illuminate how the participants in this research embodied and performed such norms. I consider what it means for abjection to be embodied, understood, lived, and felt as one's own.

This discussion of the interiority of abjection—of the move from a constitutive outside to an inside—is primarily framed through the ways in which the participants in this research pathologised and disavowed their disabled subjectivity. I draw upon ten participants in this study to illuminate the movement between the individual and the collective, the psychic and the social: these participants are *Clifton Murphy, Richard Brady, Joshua Rodgers, Jake Hawkins, Lisa Austin, Anne-Marie Holloway, Amal Alam, Peter Camilleri, Freddie Watkins*, and *Roger Cobb*.[1] The tropes of pathologisation and disavowal emerged through a discursive and narrative analysis of the thirteen life histories, and are discussed through the theoretical framing of

Foucault's (1972, 1978, 1980) account of the constitutive power of discourse (discussed previously in Chapter 1 and outlined in the Appendix).

This account of discourse is considered alongside the social and psychic approach to abjection I develop in this book. It is also important to point out that while I work with individual narratives in this chapter, I do so in order to highlight that 'any single account of experience is always an account of other times, places, subjects and practices' (Bansel 2012: 7). In this way I position the participants' individual accounts of experience as more than individual; rather, they are socially constituted and in turn constitute one's psychic life. I therefore foreground the continuities and repetitions across the participants' life history narratives (and subsequently, my analysis of them), for each of the stories shows how prevailing discourses and practices of ableism and disablism inform the sense their narrators make of their own lives.

In so doing, I address the ways in which the narratives of disabled people who participated in this research illuminate how they variously regulate, resist, or reproduce the different technologies and discourses through which their subject positions have been constituted and embodied. Two main questions guide this enquiry: *how do disabled people embody abjection, and what are the psychic and material effects of this embodiment?* Addressing these questions illuminates both the practices through which dis/ability is produced and embodied and the embodied/material effects of these practices. Here, I theorise how discourses of pathologisation and disavowal can illuminate the ways in which social practices constitute the psychic life of the subject through the embodiment and performance of normative, ableist discourses. Further, pathologisation and disavowal provide an analytical frame for exploring the ways in which participants abjected themselves.

Pathologisation

The institution of abledness is so pervasive that disability is marked as 'other' (McRuer 2006). The belief that disability is an ontological, biomedical condition is so ubiquitous that alternative conceptions are devalued, dismissed, and, in many cases, invisibilised. The hegemonic discourse that disability is a biological abnormality is so ingrained that other accounts are largely foreclosed. It is perhaps to be expected that nearly every participant in this research constructed their disabled subjectivity as abnormal and pathological. Mason (1992: 27) writes,

[i]nternalised oppression is not the cause of our mistreatment, it is the result of our mistreatment. It would not exist without the real external oppression that forms the social climate in which we exist. Once oppression has been internalised, little force is needed to keep us submissive. We harbour inside ourselves the pain and the memories, the fears and the confusions, the negative self images and the low expectations, turning them into weapons with which to re-injure ourselves, every day of our lives.

Mason (1992) illuminates here how social practices work their way into the psychic life of those who are oppressed. The focus of this chapter is not the relationships the participants have with others (discussed in the previous chapters), but the relationships they have with themselves, which is articulated as the psychic dimension of abjection. In so doing, I expose the essentialism that operates in our culture, and illuminate how normative practices become embodied and performed by the participants in this research, and the ways in which these normative practices can lead to the disavowal of disabled subjectivity.

Disavowal

The concept, and practice, of disavowal has been under-explored and under-theorised, except arguably in the realm of psychoanalysis. It broadly refers to the repudiation, rejection, or minimisation of something and, in the context of this research, I take it to mean the disavowal of disabled subjectivity. Paradoxically and simultaneously, however, disavowal also constitutes subjectivity: a 'radical refusal to identify suggests that on some level an identification has already taken place, an identification has been made and disavowed' (Butler 1997b: 149). This suggests that disabled people must acknowledge their disabled subjectivity in order to disavow it. Campbell (2009a: 25) recognises this as a double bind that entraps disabled people:

> [i]n order to attain the benefit of a 'disabled identity' one must constantly participate in the processes of disability disavowal, aspire towards the norm, reach a state of near-ablebodiedness, or at the very least to effect a state of 'passing'.

As the participants' narratives explored in this chapter demonstrate, disabled people embody and perform the idea that disability is shameful. Further, in striving for the norm, they perform various technologies/practices that work to disavow their disabled subjectivity, and embody social practices that constitute one's psychic life. In this sense, abjection operates as a regulatory norm in which disabled people must expel, minimise, or repudiate that which 'disturbs identity, system, order' (Kristeva 1982: 4). Simultaneously, then, the very disavowal of disability creates another form of abjection that re-instantiates ability/disability, normal/abnormal binaries.

A note about binaries

As I make clear in the forthcoming sections, many of the participants re-instantiated binaries of self/other, disabled/abled, normal/abnormal, and so on. One of my aims throughout this chapter is to prise open these binary constructions, and to explore the conditions in which one part of the dualism—the abled and the normal—is implicated in the oppression of the (disabled) other. As Goodley (2011: 104) writes, '[i]n order to speak of *I* (able), I must distinguish it from an *other* (disabled)'. The 'logic of identity' (Young 1990) creates dichotomous hierarchical oppositions such as good/ bad, normal/abnormal, man/woman, mind/body, and so on. These dualisms become so ingrained that their 'naturalness' goes unquestioned. Cartesian dyads situate the former category as the norm, and the latter as the opposite. The problem, however, is that the norm goes unquestioned and uninterrogated, while the deviant categories are made visible through their constant reiteration and surveillance as abnormal. In this chapter I work with the life history narratives in ways that prise open these binaries and illuminate how both the norm and its opposite are fictive constructions. I do this through attention to the accounts of experience given by the life histories of the ten participants included in this chapter.

Clifton Murphy

I interviewed *Clifton Murphy* on four occasions, and at the start of our first interview together, I asked him to tell me a little about himself:

> I was never meant to be, because I was a, what you call a love child or a mistake, my parents didn't want children, right. Um, parents lived an elaborate life of smoking, drinking, and, you know, whatever, which caused my so-called disability. I did have a brother and a sister before me but they were terminated at birth. Um, nature kept me going, so I come out damaged, right hand side cerebral palsy, um, a bit of an int-, here we go this word, intellectual disability. And I was rejected from day one.

There were a number of participants who stuttered over the term 'intellectual disability' (Clifton, Anne-Marie, Joshua, and Lisa), perhaps an indication of the social anxieties disability evokes (Shildrick 2009), and how it works on and into subjects' psychic fears. Clifton spoke more about his upbringing:

> I had a brother and sister, they were terminated, and then they tried to terminate me and it didn't work—nature brought me along. All damaged but still I was born. Then they had to make up for the damaged one so they had another one, which is my brother.

Clifton's reference to nature is complex; on the one hand, he says he comes from nature, yet, on the other, he says he is neither natural nor normal.

During our fourth interview, I asked him about his description of himself as 'damaged':

> Yeah. Why lie? I am damaged...Well, normal I believe is a person like you. You got two good arms, two good legs, you, you got a good brain,

you know. You, you talk well. That's normal. Where damaged means that, got cerebral palsy. I'm not really smart because no one took the time to help me educate…And yes, I am damaged. I can't lie about it… you've got to be honest with yourself, you're damaged…Yes, you can act like a, a, a normal person, but you're only fooling yourself, you know what I mean? You're playing a game, you know what I mean? I hate playing games.

Clifton constructs this question as a matter of honesty, and articulates the truth of himself as 'damaged'. When asked to imagine how his life could be different, Clifton replied:

Well, I'd like to have a fair go and be normal. I'd like to have all my faculties and live a normal life, you know, like everyone else. Yeah.

Clifton draws upon the dominant discourse that disability equals deficiency, and he embodies it, giving an account of himself that shows how he is inter-pellated into social norms that constitute his psychic life. The workings of scientific classification have subjectified Clifton as disabled, as a subject whose 'impairment' is understood to be real, objective, and true. Clifton conceives disability as a strictly ontological fact. He thinks that there is some-thing wrong with his body. He conceptualises disability through the lens of ab/normality, and he cites intelligence as a key marker of dis/ability. While he seems to embody the 'fact' he has a non-normative body, he nevertheless desires a normative one. In this way, Clifton acknowledges himself to be abject or outside the normative framework, and perceives these categories to be fixed, unchangeable, and unavailable to him.

Clifton's construction of his disabled subjectivity links with Oliver's (1996: 32) description of the personal tragedy theory of disability, which he defines as 'some terrible chance event which occurs at random to unfortunate individuals'. Disability, under this discourse, is understood to be ontologic-ally real and intolerable, and as Campbell (2015: 109) suggests, the 'truth games' that 'surround disability are dependent on discourses of ableism for their very legitimation'. Clifton's refusal to 'lie' suggests an investment in shoring up the stability of ableism and the abjection/pathologisation of the 'ontologically real' status of disability.

While none of the other participants explicitly spoke of the 'wrongness' of their disabled subjectivity in the same way as Clifton, they still adopted pathological discourses to talk about themselves. Interestingly, some of the participants only revealed their perception of their disabled subjectivity when they spoke about other, non-disabled people (Joshua, Jake, Peter, Lisa, Anne-Marie, and Amal). Alternatively, other participants invoked pathological discourses when they compared themselves to other disabled people (Freddie and Peter). These discourses of pathology often emerged through verbal 'slips', where revelations that were originally tangential to the topic under investigation emerged. The hegemonic assumption that disability equals deficiency and inability is so ingrained that many of the participants spoke about what was 'wrong', perhaps without realising they were doing so. These 'slips' reveal the subtle and insidious acts of abjection that suffuse the disabled body. This may illuminate the simultaneity of psychic and social lives, demonstrating how attitudes are embodied, taken in, and then expunged into the social world through 'slips'.

Richard Brady

In my second interview with *Richard Brady*, he explained to me how abled people treated him badly, which he perceived was because of his disabled subjectivity. I then asked him how he felt about disability, and he pathologised his disabled subjectivity when he spoke in terms of disability:

> Um, I don't look at my disability.
> (Mhm)
> I look at, uh, I've got ability to do things…I look beyond the disability.
> (Mhm)
> You know, it's important to me to work with my disability in a good way, not a bad way…And I look at the positive side of it, not the negative side of it, where I might be able to do things but, hey, let's have a go…it's important to show people that you can do things for yourself, and improve yourself, and that's what I like to do…Now I say people first, disability second.

Richard draws on a contemporary political discourse available in disability culture that encourages disabled people to focus on their ability rather than their disability (Siebers 2008). The personification of this discourse would be the *supercrip*,[2] which Grue (2015) refers to as a disabled figure who is afforded attention and recognition when they 'achieve' something *in spite of* their disability. This is based on the presumption that disabled people are incapable of achieving anything and, as such, are constituted as exceptional when able to do something (Clare 2015; Grue 2015, 2016). Clare (2015: 2) provides the following examples:

> [a] boy without hands bats .486 on his Little League team. A blind man hikes the Appalachian Trail from end to end. An adolescent girl with Down syndrome learns to drive and has a boyfriend. A guy with one leg runs across Canada.

While these stories evoke marvel and wonder, they do not address the underlying conditions in which 'it is so difficult for people with Down syndrome to have romantic partners, for blind people to have adventures, for disabled kids to play sports' (Clare 2015: 2–3). To focus on what disabled people can do merely reinforces the 'superior' able body/mind (Clare 2015).

Richard is suggesting that there is something negative about disability and that one must, in Richard's words, 'improve yourself' to reach the abled norm. Yet Richard's description also points to resistance; he does not want to strip away disability completely, but rather conceives it as something extra to his own view of the world. Richard also subscribes to the binary logic, foregrounding his desire to be 'good' and 'positive' rather than 'bad' and 'negative'. His desire to 'do things' corresponds with popular conceptions of disability as an inability to do things (Titchkosky 2007), and Richard seeks to 'do things' to resist attitudes towards disability.

In the above exchange Richard also says he subscribes to 'people first' language (that is, 'people with disability'), which brings into question the humanness of disabled bodies:

> [p]erson-first language is typically used to emphasize personhood, as well as the conditionality of disability, and the idea that disability and persons ought to be separate. The political efficacy of stating, 'We are people too,' is questionable since it asserts, 'I am the type of person that you may not imagine as fully human'.
>
> (Titchkosky 2007: 196)

This taking up of person-first language foregrounds the extent to which a *people first* discourse suggests that the humanness of disabled people is debatable in the first place. As Hughes (2007: 677–678) writes, '[w]hen people feel that they have to make a claim to humanity they are usually already in big trouble'. As I have suggested earlier, this form of abjection brings disabled bodies into the 'shadowy regions of ontology' (Butler, in Meijer and Prins 1998: 277). The negation of disabled ontologies works to negate and erase the (disabled) subject's formation.

In trying to attain the (abled) norm, and focussing on privileging ability and minimising disability, I suggest that Richard is also invested in disavowing his disabled subjectivity. This interpretation is informed by an example from my own queer life. During my PhD, on a Friday, I would go to a pub near university campus with a few other PhD candidates. We drank beer, played pool, engaged in banter, and tried to forget our PhD struggles. The pub is in an industrial area in the western suburbs of Sydney; distinctly working-class, men wear hi-vis workwear[3] and 'bikini waitresses' serve drinks after 4 pm. As a gay man, I understand that this pub is 'not for me', and this leaves me feeling very queer in a non-queer place. Perhaps this articulation of queerness means that I am stereotyping everyone there, but I feel that I need to check my behaviour. When I (sometimes try to) performatively embody heterosexuality, I cannot avoid disavowing my queer subjectivity.

Likewise, when Richard foregrounds ability, he is disavowing disability. I speculate that this is a strategic decision through which Richard disarms the damaging effects of 'disability' (like I do with 'queerness'), and yet this still has negative consequences for the category of disability (and, for me, queerness). The binary emerges again when Richard articulates that it is better to overcome than succumb to disability. Paradoxically, as Richard and I disavow our subjectivities, the message appears to be that one must be as (hetero)normatively abled as possible. In our complex embodiments and performances, we simultaneously highlight the fluid and agentic nature of our identities, along with our sense that we are outside the norm.

On another occasion Richard said,

> I always tell people when I give, give a talk 'You all got a disability as well as me. We mightn't see yours, but you see mine'…we all have a disability in one way or another.

By trying to highlight the pervasiveness of disability, Richard is invested here in disavowing any totalising account of his disabled subjectivity. While it is a strategic device that he uses to alleviate negative attitudes towards disability, it is still a disablist practice. You do not often hear people proclaim, '*We are all gay in one way or another,*' or '*We are all black in one way or another,*' to justify one's subjectivity. Richard's actions are a technology that he deploys because he recognises the oppressive attitudes society places upon disability, yet the varied nature with which he disavows disability also points to his own agency. Perhaps his strategy is a technology that is only available to disabled people (and queer people), where ability (and heterosexuality) are arguably temporary/malleable subjectivities. It may be that Richard's strategy is to highlight abled people's precarity in order to promote the idea that abledness (and heterosexuality) is just as constructed as disability.

Joshua Rodgers

Like Richard, *Joshua Rodgers* pathologised his disabled subjectivity when he spoke in relation to abled people. He compared himself to abled people who he called 'normal people'. In this sense, he has 'othered' himself in simply making this distinction. When I interviewed Joshua, he told me his sister was non-disabled, and consequently 'pretty lucky'. This again mirrors the personal tragedy theory of disability, whereby disability occurs through chance, misfortune, or lottery. At another point in our interviews, he spoke about another person, and after I asked if they were disabled, he replied 'no, he seemed normal'. In both instances Joshua compares himself to abled people and situates his disabled subjectivity as abnormal. It could be progressive/radical for Joshua to say that he is 'not normal', but by saying that one is lucky to be abled, he positions disability as an inferior, unlucky, and abject state.

On another occasion Joshua simply said he had something 'wrong with me', and when he spoke of disability he said,

> people with disability are just normal people that have something [pause] extra maybe, or, I don't want to say a fault, because you've got to look at what they can do not what they can't do.

Here Joshua conceptualises disability as something that is added to one's embodiment (which could be positive), yet something that is a 'fault'. There are several similarities between Richard and Joshua's accounts of disability, and as I mentioned earlier, it is noteworthy to highlight that they are father and son. When Joshua focusses on what one 'can' do rather than what one 'cannot' do, he mirrors Richard's disavowal of disability and the privileging of the supercrip. Like Richard, Joshua also deploys person-first terminology. This person-first speech naturalises the experience of specific forms of embodiment (abject or otherwise):

> [t]he 'naturalness' of the notion of the able-bodied liberal individual coupled with the negation of a disabled sensibility makes many disabled people queue for the chance to be anointed as 'people first', while simultaneously disavowing their previous embodied positions as 'gimps' and 'cripples'. Ironically, disabled people who achieve 'people first' status are not achieving full normative status but are only legitimizing an able-bodied resemblance through their desire for normality.
>
> (Overboe 1999: 24)

Overboe (1999) goes on to suggest that this pursuit creates a continuum, ranging from *successful* 'people first' disabled people, to pitiful 'gimps' and 'cripples' deemed worthless. In any event, as I illuminate in this chapter, disabled people embody normative discourses about disability as they are invested in privileging the abled subject by pathologising their own embodiment. This is made possible through the normative discourses and practices through which they come to understand that a disabled body is negative, incapable, and worthless:

> [o]ne need only consider the way in which the history of having been called an injurious name is embodied, how the words enter the limbs, craft the gesture, bend the spine...how these slurs accumulate over time, dissimulating their history, taking on the semblance of the natural, configuring and restricting the *doxa* that counts as 'reality'.
>
> (Butler 1997a: 159, italics in original)

Butler (1997a: 159) calls this the 'carry[ing of] the mnemic trace of the body', which represents the movement from the psychic to the social, interior to the exterior, repeatedly and cyclically. Joshua, influenced by an ableist world—and his own father—learns and understands that disability is negative and inferior, and that the social practices through which disability is constituted have worked their way into the psychic dimensions of Joshua, moving simultaneously from the collective to the individual, from the social to the psychic.

Jake Hawkins

When speaking about his experience of work, *Jake Hawkins* pathologised his disabled subjectivity. In his account, the ab/normal dyad was also evident:

> Oh, um, at the moment I'm doing work placements...the last work placements before these one's, my disability got in the way because a) I had to actually be told twice what to do, and, like, 'cause, with, with my disability, like a normal person has to be told once what to do, but I have to be told twice, or maybe shown how to do it. Otherwise, like, I wouldn't know what to do, so yeah.

In this remark Jake compares himself to normal people and suggests there is something delimiting about disability. Interestingly, he also describes disability as something that 'gets in the way', contrasting with Joshua's suggestion that it is something 'added' to one's embodiment. The spatiality of abjection is exposed where Jake and Joshua suggest it is something that can be navigated beyond, beneath, or beside. Also, when Jake says that 'normal people' only need to be told 'once what to do', I suggest that Jake has a fantastical idea of the normal body, what Lorde (1984: 116) calls the 'mythical norm'.

The norm is rarely scrutinised, and disabled people are so often (over-) studied, marked, and defined that the 'normal body' is presented in mythical perfection, while the disabled body is described as lacking and deficient (Goodley 2014). Davis (1995: 24), in acknowledging this dilemma, suggests that 'the "problem" is not the person with disabilities; the problem is the way that normalcy is constructed to create the "problem" of the disabled person'. Jake extends this comparison to abled people:

> Like sometimes, sometimes it's hard because you don't know what they're gonna like, react to you, 'cause you have a disability and they don't. They don't actually know what you've been through in your l-, like, your life. 'Cause, they, um, they would have their life as perfect as they can, but, um, you would have your disability that restricts you from, um, from living your life how you want to. And that, um, if you don't, like in my case if I didn't have the disability, my life would be different, but like, unfortunately I've got the disability, I just put up with it. But, like, I've faced it like, it's a disability I'll have for the rest of my life, I'm not worried, people think different, they can. I couldn't care, so yeah.

Again, Jake compares himself to abled people and, through this, marks himself as inferior. He seems to construct disability as self-restricting, rather than looking at how society restricts disabled bodies.

At the start of his explanation, he also creates some distance between his position as a disabled subject instead referring to what other disabled people are like and how they would strive for perfection in the face of restriction. Yet he is at the same time talking about himself, and towards the end of this dialogue, he re-assumes his position as a disabled subject when he talks about 'I' and disability. It may be the case that Jake finds it unpalatable to directly reference himself as a disabled subject when he talks of external restrictions that limit his agency, or 'from living your life how you want to'. Towards the end of his monologue, he retakes his position in abjection but only to suggest it is 'unfortunate' he has a disability. Mirroring the personal tragedy theory of disability, he perceives of his disability as a matter of chance or lottery. As it is something Jake says he must 'put up with', he resigns himself to his disabled subjectivity and suggests he does not care what other people may think of him. And yet, in order to *not care*, Jake must have at some stage made the assessment about whether it is worth caring about.

Lisa Austin

Like Jake, *Lisa Austin* compared her disabled subjectivity to abled people:

> So I'm counting my lucky stars that [Stephanie[4]] is not disabled. In some ways I wish she was, 'cause it might bring up more to have a better chance 'cause I know what to do with children that are disabled. I know about the, getting the, getting the early intervention. I know about trying to educate them early 'cause they don't forget it. But, you know, at the same time, I'll never wish my worst enemy to have a disability unless it's, you know, it can't be helped.

Again, 'luck' is referenced as the source, and she presumes disability as an unlucky chance event that 'can't be helped'. Signifying her abhorrence to a disabled subjectivity, for Lisa, disability is constructed as so terrible that she would not want even her worst enemy to be disabled. She continued:

> it's sad in a way, my, I think it's a really nice thing but my ex-mother-in-law says 'Well if you look at her [Stephanie], you see both of your parents, just without the disabilities'. I go 'Wow, that's nice'. And then I look at her and go 'I wish I was like you now'. And then that makes me a little bit sad that I've even got it, and, but you know I can't change that, so. I think, well, then I go back to thinking 'Well I wish I was like that'. And maybe I can watch her and I can learn something else that will get me a little closer to like that. But, you know, anyway.

Lisa's abjection has been compounded; she acknowledges her disability, and this puts her in a further state of sadness:

in a way it's sad I didn't get that normal 'cause, I can't do what I wanted to do, but then I think, well if I was normal, then I wouldn't be sitting where I am now.

Ability is prized, and disability devalued, by both Lisa and her ex-mother-in-law. The constant references to 'normal' situate disability, and Lisa, as abnormal. There is also a shifting desire in what Lisa has articulated; on one hand, she fantasises about having a disabled daughter because she is disabled, and on the other, she wishes she was non-disabled because her daughter is 'normal'. This is a complex and contradictory position to take. As abjection works as a regulatory norm, Lisa is disavowing her capacity to be a mother if she does not 'fall' within the same dis/abled identity as her daughter.

On another occasion Lisa pathologised her disabled subjectivity in more general ways. Lisa simply said she was not normal; she said,

> I guess it's different and it's just hard 'cause you feel like you're almost like, whatever they wanna call 'normal'. But then you know you're not, so. But, you know, so, but anyway.

Here, Lisa explicitly says she is abnormal, constructing the binary of dis/ability as a question of ab/normality. I argue that it is fully legitimate and healthy to claim abnormality. However, when this abnormality is tied to luck, or the desire to be abled, there is a risk that pathological discourses constitute embodiment. In embodying disablist and ableist discourses, the individual is constituted as both 'other' and 'abject'.

Anne-Marie Holloway

Anne-Marie Holloway compared herself to abled people specifically in relation to distinctions between herself and me: between disability and temporary abledness. As I discuss more fully in Chapter 7, Anne-Marie was discriminated against by the police when she reported domestic violence. She outlines her interaction with the police thus:

> They're meant to help us, but they don't know how to deal with people in the community. See 'cause if you go to the police, they're gonna, they're gonna, um, like, listen to you more because you don't have a problem, and I think they judge us that have an intellectual disability. And I suppose if someone else has got a mental, uh, mental health issue it could be very confuse for the police to work it out. But they're putting people with an intellectual disability all in one category.

In this exchange, Anne-Marie told me that I—a temporarily abled man—did not have a 'problem', and in doing so, indicates that she sees (her) disabled subjectivity as a problem or problematic. Like Peter and Jake, Anne-Marie re-instantiates a binary logic, where disabled people have problems and abled people do not. Anne-Marie's assumption that abled people do not have problems—in whatever kind of capacity—is again a mythic notion (Lorde 1984). The abjection of certain bodies, and the lack of interrogation of the norm, creates the impression that abled people are perfect while disabled people are deficient, abnormal, and imperfect. This behoves us to consider more seriously the lives of different bodies in all their forms, and to promote difference and varied/alternative forms of embodiment (Goodley and Runswick-Cole 2013; Mitchell, Snyder, and Ware 2014). I return to Anne-Marie's life history narrative more fully in Chapter 7.

Amal Alam

Amal Alam compared herself to abled people in much more general terms. As I mentioned earlier, Amal is blind, and she experiences people walking up to her on the street and asking rude questions about the nature of her disability, such as whether she will ever have a family, and if she has any money to hand out. In this sense, people assume to know something of the psychic dimension of Amal, whereby her desires are read as normatively similar to theirs (abled people) and unachievable because of her perceived disability ('will you ever have a family?'). Abled people may believe disabled people have different desires, and if they share similar desires, a sense of disorientation occurs. This illuminates how psychic presumptions work their way into social contexts and environments.

In any event, sometimes Amal finds these questions rude and sometimes not, and this is mediated by the context and nature of the questions. In response to that which she considers rude, Amal said,

> Mm, like, I think it's not right, just because I have something wrong with me, you shouldn't look at me in the wrong way. You should treat me as a normal person.

Amal cites the 'wrongness' of her body as the source of people's rudeness towards her. She appears to accept that she is different compared to abled people, and she embodies these differences as an abnormal and negative trait. There is also a tension here in Amal's desires; she oscillates between saying she is abnormal/wrong and wanting to be treated as a 'normal person'. Perhaps Amal sees no reason why her disabled subjectivity should cause disablist treatment from others?

During our third interview Amal made a reference to 'normal people', so I asked her if she considered herself 'not normal':

> No. I, I see my, um, I see myself, um, with my disability I'm still normal to act and communicate and talk to people—I'm not that severe disability.

As Overboe (1999) describes, Amal has created a continuum of disability, where 'mild intellectual disability' is constituted as not as 'severe' as others. Amal has drawn a distinction in order to minimise her own disability, thus pathologising and disavowing her own (disabled) subjectivity. In comparing herself to more abject others, Amal has also abjected herself by expelling what she finds intolerable about herself (Kristeva 1982), illustrating her agency and power to abjectify others.

Peter Camilleri

Like Amal's comparisons between disability and abledness, *Peter Camilleri* also spoke about his interactions with these embodiments/subjectivities. In this exchange, he both pathologises and disavows his disabled subjectivity when he states that he sometimes does not disclose his disability:

Yeah I just, I just make out that there's nothing wrong with me.

(Yeah, and how do you do that?)

Just do normal things, like you're supposed to, not do like, a person with a disability does.

It is unclear what Peter does in order to leave the impression that he is abled. Yet Peter suggests that there is something 'wrong' with disabled people, and when he says he tries to act normally, he implicitly recognises there is something abnormal about how disabled people behave. His mention of acting the way 'you're supposed to' also highlights that standards of behaviour and conduct are socially imposed, and it forecloses different forms of behaviour and embodiment that disabled people should be able to express (see Garland Thomson 1996; Goodley 2013; Goodley and Runswick-Cole 2013; Shildrick 2015, 2002). Whereas Clifton is invested in the 'truth' of his 'damage', Peter is interested in concealing/disavowing such damaging truth and performatively embodying abledness. On another occasion Peter said he 'put[s] it [disability] behind me', which is yet another example of his disavowal of disability and of his practice of expelling that which is abject.

Peter again pathologises his disabled subjectivity when he tells me how others react to the disclosure of his disability:

They just go into shock.

(Go into shock?)

Yeah, like they couldn't, they can't believe that I've got something wrong.

Peter's reference that disabled people have something 'wrong' with them counterpoises the idea that non-disabled people have something 'right' with them. Again, similar to Richard, Jake, Lisa, and Anne-Marie, there is a re-instantiation of a binary logic, where disabled people automatically have something wrong with them compared to the 'right' non-disabled body. The re-instantiation of these binary constructions reinforces existing power structures that render disabled people inferior and non-normative.

On another occasion, Peter pathologised his disabled subjectivity in relation to other disabled people. He said:

> Like some people they can't move their arms and that, but I can move mine and that, and when I see people like that you sort of, makes me upset that they can't have normal feelings in their arms and that.

Here Peter implicitly highlights the non-normative and abnormal position of disabled people. Moreover, he indicates that 'normal' can be applied to different parts of the body (arms, for example), rather than the whole person or subject. It is unclear what kinds of bodily movements he privileges over others. Nevertheless, he abjectifies those with physical disability to preserve his own bodily integrity, yet simultaneously acknowledges the abnormality of disability in general. Peter has created hierarchies of disability, and he abjectifies physically disabled people who do not have 'normal feelings in their arms'.

On another occasion, when talking about disabled people generally, Peter said,

> Um, I feel sorry for them, the way they are. And, that they can do, fend for themselves, and get around. And some of them can't. Sometimes I feel sorry, yeah.

By not self-identifying as 'some of them [who] can't', Peter is abjectifying his own disability and vacating the present ('I just put it behind me'); he feels sorry for other disabled people as if he is not similarly constituted as such. Perhaps Peter found it unpalatable to talk about himself as a disabled person. In any event, throughout these exchanges, he continually distances himself from disabled subjectivity, disavowing it and abjectifying himself in the process.

Freddie Watkins

Freddie Watkins also pathologised (his) disabled subjectivity in relation to other disabled people. Initially, he did not see himself as being different, saying,

> I don't class myself as being different to them [abled people].

Yet he then went on to say,

even though I've got the disability, I'm not, I don't have the real bad disability. I've only got it mildly, 'Cause a lot of people can't function, or do things for themselves.

(Yep)

…and I can. And that's where a lot of people are different to me.

In this exchange, Freddie implicitly highlights the indignity of being disabled—according to normative social processes—and seeks to highlight that *his disability* is not severe. Through this process, he pathologises disability.

Freddie also presents disability as a continuum, where some forms of disabled subjectivity are considered worse than others. As Overboe (1999) described, Freddie may see others as part of different sub-groups of disabilities and hierarchise different forms of disability. Baynton (2001) suggests that the historical oppression of other abjected groups has been justified by constituting such groups as disabled. For example, queer lives are often framed by notions of biological or psychological abnormalities, women with physical/intellectual/psychological flaws, and racial and religious minorities with disease (see Baynton 2001; Gilman 1991, for example). This leads Siebers (2008: 6) to suggest that disability 'marks the last frontier of unbridled inferiority'. Freddie's sentiments illustrate how such discourses about disability have become embodied and performed, and that even disabled people are invested in disavowing disabled subjectivities. Freddie abjects other disabled people, but he also abjectifies himself because he casts out that which he perceives to be intolerable in himself and on to bodies that he constitutes as more abject. Through this process, Freddie simultaneously subjects others to his idea of 'normal' and embodies discourses of ableism.

Roger Cobb

Roger Cobb also constructed his disabled subjectivity in damaging ways. Earlier I described Roger's experience of rape. When we spoke about this experience, I asked him why he thought the man had targeted him; he replied:

Well, I'm sure it was because of my disability. Because that person saw that I could be, you know, a bit slow with something, I don't know. There's something different about me.

Roger suggests he is 'slow' intellectually, and that he is different to most other people. Notwithstanding the fact that all people go through changes concerning intellectual development throughout their lives, these differences are taken to only apply, and to only matter, to disabled people (Titchkosky 2007).

Roger also suggests he is 'different', and while difference may certainly be embraced, during this exchange it was clear to me that Roger was talking about difference in a reductive and negative sense. On another occasion, Roger also appears to suggest that disability is a question of in/sanity. He says:

> Until this very day I still don't see myself as a person with an intellectual disability. I'm a normal, or whatever normal is, I'm a, I'm as sane as the person next door.

The binaries are present here again, where Roger seems to suggest that disability is a question of ab/normality, and that disabled people are insane while abled people are sane. It is unclear where or why Roger draws upon the claim that intellectual disability is entangled with questions of in/sanity. It may be that Roger has conflated intellectual disability and mental health, a common practice that is evidenced in the wider literature (see, for example, Arneil 2009; Hall and Kearns 2001). It may also be that Roger's treatment as a disabled subject has actually precipitated his mental health issues. He may be conflating the two constructs because he sees them as compatible or causational.

While above he spoke about in/sanity, later he took a different approach. He said,

> Well I believe that everyone's got a disability, OK. Mine is that I've got glasses. [His partner] is that she smokes. [His support worker] is that, um, she had a, a, an illness that could have taken her life. Um, yeah. [pause] I've had, yeah, OK. I don't think anyone's got, I believe everyone's got a disability, but I don't see why we have to go around with that label on our shoulder.

On another occasion, he similarly stated,

> I believe that I do not have a disability. I believe that the only thing that makes me different to you is I wear glasses and you don't. You've got a pen in your hand, I don't. You're drinking water, I'm drinking coffee. I'm being silly...I believe that everybody on this earth has a disability of some kind.

Roger's comments raise several important considerations. He highlights the pernicious effects of labelling, which often re-instantiate negative perceptions of difference. Why would someone want to be a member of a group which is ubiquitously oppressed? Simultaneously, then, Roger is trying to disarm 'disability' of its damaging political power, yet this very process is an admission that there is something 'wrong' or devalued about disability. Roger seeks to minimise his disability by simultaneously highlighting its pervasiveness across society, thus rejecting the labelling of some populations and not others.

Whereas Richard earlier disavowed his disabled subjectivity as a strategic option, in these passages, Roger may do so as a defensive condition of possibility because he finds being labelled threatening (and for good reason given that his life history illustrates that this threat is justified). Roger further extends his point:

> Why label people? You know, we've had labels all our lives, pills shoved down our throats, been told you're gotta do this, you're gotta do that, you're gotta do this, oh, for fuck's sake! When can we just start living a normal life? You know, why do we have to have a label? Do you have a label?
>
> (I don't know)[5]
>
> I don't think you would.

Roger is aware that the disability label is damaging (in contrast to the other labels he mentions), as he has been labelled most of his life in institutional settings. It is a recognition he seeks to repudiate and resist.

Pathologisation and disavowal *considered*

I have explored the ways in which abjection moves from the social body to the individual body, how it moves into the self and out again as it is cast out and onto the bodies of others. I have also explored the ways in which many of the participants in this research have pathologised and disavowed their disabled subjectivity. They have done so, I suggest, because of the pervasive ableism and disablism that tells them that a disabled subjectivity is undesirable and abject. They have embodied and performed normative and essentialist understandings of disability, where their embodiment is perceived in relation to a naturalised and ontological condition. They have embodied and performed discourses that infer there is something wrong and abnormal about their embodiment, and that it must be disavowed because the normal body is constituted as the fully human body.

Given that abjection works as a regulatory norm (Butler 1993; Tyler 2013), my imperative in this chapter has been to expose and critique the normative assumptions about disabled bodies, and the ways in which the participants embodied these discourses and pathologised their own disabled subjectivity. At the same time, it was not my intention to *criticise* these participants for constructing their subjectivity through discourses of pathology and abnormality. Given the ableism that pervades society, it would have been remarkable if they did not embody, nor draw upon, these pathologising discourses to describe themselves and their experiences (Campbell 2008, 2009a, 2009b; Goodley 2014; McRuer 2006). As Lotringer (as cited in Tyler

2013: 43) writes, '[p]eople don't just become abject because they are treated like a thing, but because they become a thing to themselves'. My aim is to highlight the abjected positions through which disabled subjects are constituted, and, at the same time, argue for alternative ways in which disability can be thought of and constituted in public discourse.

In critiquing normative discourses and practices, I also emphasise that it is not automatically negative to actively embody and embrace difference. I, for one, acknowledge my difference as a queer man, and am proud of it. Thus, when the disabled participants in this research have said that they are different, I do not necessarily assume that they are pathologising their (disabled) subjectivity. Rather, I have made the claim that they are pathologising their disabled subjectivity in instances when they themselves claim they are different *in a negative, reductive, or pathological sense.* In the context of gender, Clare (2015: xxviii) writes,

> I want my gendered story to be one of many stories that defy, bend, smash the gender binary. But in the end, what I really want is for all the many gendered possibilities in the world to be, not normal, but rather profoundly ordinary and familiar.

Clare's (2015) desire might be understood as a 'passionate attachment' to being a transgressive (gendered) subject, and that 'there is no formation of the subject without a passionate attachment to [this] subjection' (Butler 1997b: 67). Bansel (2008: 164) suggests that passionate attachment derives 'in part from our dependency on technologies, practices and discourses that instantiate and sustain our desire to "be", and to be recognised'. Passionate attachments make up one's psychic life, and to appropriate Clare's (2015) desire, I am passionately attached to the possibility that disabled people might come to embrace their disability and find possibilities to be not normal, but rather profoundly ordinary and familiar. I revisit this attachment to reimagining disabled subjectivities later in the book, along with possibilities to disrupt and resist the ability/disability, normal/abnormal binaries through which disabled subjects are constituted as other.

According to Cartesian dualisms, disability is constructed as abnormal while ability becomes the norm. As there is so much emphasis on the other (disability), the first and privileged half of the binary (ability) is uninterrogated. In line with Greenstein's (2016: 29) conceptualisation, I suggest that ability is just as fantastical, and just as constructed, as disability:

> [o]nce we understand disability not as a trait tied to an individual body or mind but as a socially created binary, it is impossible to claim that only one side of the binary (the disabled) is socially constructed, while the other (the 'normal') is a natural or neutral position.

While ability and disability are both performatively constituted and embodied, the participants in this research, like most people, perceive them to be naturally occurring. Indeed, the disabled participants in this research constructed their subjectivity in relation to the idea of the norm: the abled person.

Siebers (2008) and Titchkosky (2003, 2007) have argued that disability is often conceptualised as an inability to do things, and the more someone is unable to do something, the less human they become. Butler (2004: 2) writes,

> [c]ertain humans are recognized as less than human, and that form of qualified recognition does not lead to a viable life. Certain humans are not recognized as human at all.

Many disabled people experience and embody this belief by abjecting themselves and others. They may feel that there is little option but to recognise the 'deficiency' of their bodies, and to disavow it at all costs. Disabled people are not granted the status of subjects; their attempts to re-write the subjective accounts of disability are inefficacious because their disavowal does not do the work that disavowing is meant to do; instead it becomes another form of abjection that pathologises disability.

The unintentional pathologisation of disability and its disavowal necessitates a rethinking of the discourses surrounding dis/ability and the pervasive ableism that envelopes us. The disavowal documented in this chapter also requires us to consider how the terms of dis/ability intelligibility may be (re)imagined so that disabled people are not reduced to less than human, or their embodiment reduced to the negative attitudes that inform ableism. In the next chapter, I continue my account of the abject by considering the life history of Anne-Marie, and build upon my previous arguments to examine how abjection works in psychic and social, singular and collective dimensions, and, importantly, how abjection might possibly be resisted.

Notes

1 The narratives of Deb, Emma Silva, and Warren Goodwin are not drawn upon in this chapter because they did not pathologise or disavow their disabled subjectivity in their interviews.
2 This term shares parallels with Titchkosky's (2007) notion of the abled-disabled and Haraway's (1991) cyborg.
3 Hi-vis is short for 'high visibility'.
4 Lisa's daughter, introduced in chapter three. Not her real name.
5 Being gay did jump to mind, but I decided not to disclose (and, hence, I disavowed).

References

Arneil, B 2009, 'Disability, Self Image, and Modern Political Theory', *Political Theory*, 37(2): 218–242.

Bansel, P 2008, *Subjectivity at Work*, unpublished PhD thesis, University of Western Sydney.

Bansel, P 2012, 'Resisting and Re/counting the Power of Number: The One in the Many and the Many in the One', in *Discourse, Power, and Resistance down Under*, edited by M Vicars, T McKenna, and J White, Sense Publishers, Rotterdam, pp. 1–8.

Baynton, DC 2001, 'Disability and the Justification of Inequality in American History', in *The New Disability History: American Perspectives*, edited by PK Longmore and L Umansky, New York University Press, New York and London, pp. 33–57.

Butler, J 1990, *Gender Trouble: Feminism and the Subversion of Identity*, Routledge, New York and London.

Butler, J 1993, *Bodies that Matter: On the Discursive Limits of 'Sex'*, Routledge, New York and London.

Butler, J 1997a, *The Psychic Life of Power: Theories in Subjection*, Stanford University Press, Stanford.

Butler, J 1997b, *Excitable Speech: A Politics of the Performative*, Routledge, New York and London.

Butler, J 2000, 'Competing Universalities', in *Contingency, Hegemony, Universality: Contemporary Dialogues on the Left*, edited by J Butler, E Laclau, and S Žižek, Verso, London and New York, pp. 136–181.

Butler, J 2004, *Undoing Gender*, Routledge, London and New York.

Campbell, FAK 2008, 'Exploring Internalized Ableism Using Critical Race Theory', *Disability & Society*, 23(2): 151–162.

Campbell, FK 2009a, *Contours of Ableism: The Production of Disability and Abledness*, Palgrave Macmillan, London and New York.

Campbell, FK 2009b, 'Disability Harms: Exploring Internalized Ableism', in *Disabilities: Insights from across Fields and around the World, Volume 1, the Experience: Definitions, Causes, and Consequences*, edited by CA Marshall, E Kendall, ME Banks, and RMS Gover, Praeger Publishers, Westport, CT, pp. 19–33.

Campbell, FK 2015, 'Legislating Disability: Negative Ontologies and the Government of Legal Identities', in *Foucault and the Government of Disability*, 2nd, edition, edited by S Tremain, University of Michigan Press, Ann Arbor, MI, pp. 108–130.

Clare, E 2015, *Exile and Pride: Disability, Queerness, and Liberation*, 16th anniversary edition, Duke University Press, Durham and London.

Davis, LJ 1995, *Enforcing Normalcy: Disability, Deafness, and the Body*, Verso, London and New York.

Foucault, M 1972, *Archaeology of Knowledge*, translated by A.M Sheridan Smith, Routledge, London.

Foucault, M 1978, *The History of Sexuality, Vol. I: An Introduction*, translated by Robert Hurley, Pantheon Books, New York.

Foucault, M 1980, 'Two Lectures', in *Power/Knowledge: Selected Interviews and Other Writings, 1972–1977*, edited by C Gordon, Harvester Press Ltd, Sussex, pp. 78–108.

Garland Thomson, R 1996, 'Introduction: From Wonder to Error—A Genealogy of Freak Discourse in Modernity', in *Freakery: Cultural Spectacles of the*

Extraordinary Body, edited by R Garland Thomson, New York University Press, New York and London, pp. 1–19.

Gilman, S 1991, *The Jew's Body*, Routledge, New York and London.

Goodley, D 2011, *Disability Studies: An Interdisciplinary Introduction*, SAGE, London.

Goodley, D 2013, 'Dis/entangling Critical Disability Studies', *Disability & Society*, 28 (5): 631–644.

Goodley, D 2014, *Dis/ability Studies: Theorising Disablism and Ableism*, Routledge, London and New York.

Goodley, D and Runswick-Cole, R 2013, 'The Body as Disability and Possability: Theorizing the "Leaking, Lacking and Excessive" Bodies of Disabled Children', *Scandinavian Journal of Disability Research*, 15(1): 1–19.

Greenstein, A 2016, *Radical Inclusive Education: Disability, Teaching and Struggles for Liberation*, Routledge, London and New York.

Grue, J 2015, 'The Problem of the Supercrip: Representation and Misrepresentation of Disability', in *Disability Research Today: International Perspectives*, edited by T Shakespeare, Routledge, London and New York, pp. 204–218.

Grue, J 2016, 'The Problem with Inspiration Porn: A Tentative Definition and A Provisional Critique', *Disability & Society*, 31(6): 838–849.

Hall, E and Kearns, R 2001, 'Making Space for the "Intellectual" in Geographies of Disability', *Health & Place*, 7(3): 237–246.

Haraway, DJ 1991, *Simians, Cyborgs, and Women: The Reinvention of Nature*, Routledge, New York.

Hughes, B 2007, 'Being Disabled: Towards a Critical Social Ontology for Disability Studies', *Disability & Society*, 22(7): 673–684.

Kristeva, J 1982, *Powers of Horror: An Essay on Abjection*, translated by LS Roudiez, Columbia University Press, New York.

Lorde, A 1984, *Sister Outsider: Essays and Speeches by Audre Lorde*, The Crossing Press, Freedom, CA.

Mason, M 1992, 'Internalised Oppression', in *Disability Equality in the Classroom: A Human Rights Issue*, edited by R Rieser and M Mason, Disability Equality in Education, London, pp. 27–28.

McRuer, R 2006, *Crip Theory: Cultural Signs of Queerness and Disability*, New York University Press, New York and London.

Meijer, IC and Prins, B (with J Butler) 1998, 'How Bodies Come to Matter: An Interview with Judith Butler', *Signs: Journal of Women in Culture and Society*, 23(2): 275–286.

Mitchell, DT, Snyder, SL, and Ware, L 2014, '"[every] Child Left Behind": Curricular Cripistemologies and the Crip/Queer Art of Failure', *Journal of Literary & Cultural Disability Studies*, 8(3): 295–313.

Oliver, M 1996, *Understanding Disability: From Theory to Practice*, Macmillan, London.

Overboe, J 1999, '"Difference in Itself": Validating Disabled People's Lived Experience', *Body & Society*, 5(4): 17–29.

Shildrick, M 2002, *Embodying the Monster: Encounters with the Vulnerable Self*, SAGE, London.

Shildrick, M 2009, *Dangerous Discourses of Disability, Subjectivity and Sexuality*, Palgrave Macmillan, Basingstoke, Hampshire.

Shildrick, M 2015, '"Why Should Our Bodies End at the Skin?": Embodiment, Boundaries, and Somatechnics', *Hypatia*, 30(1): 13–29.

Siebers, T 2008, *Disability Theory*, The University of Michigan Press, Ann Arbor, MI.

Titchkosky, T 2003, *Disability, Self, and Society*, University of Toronto Press, Toronto.

Titchkosky, T 2007, *Reading and Writing Disability Differently: The Textured Life of Embodiment*, University of Toronto Press, Toronto.

Tyler, I 2013, *Revolting Subjects: Social Abjection and Resistance in Neoliberal Britain*, Zed Books, London and New York.

Young, IM 1990, *Justice and the Politics of Difference*, Princeton University Press, Princeton, NJ.

7 Anne-Marie's narrative
Abjection and resistance

Anne-Marie is forthright and persistent, and these attributes proved instrumental in the resistance to her abjection as documented in her narrative in this chapter. In relating Deb and Roger's narratives, I focussed on the ways in which abjection has been pressed upon them by others. In the preceding chapter, I focussed on the psychic dimensions of abjection where it becomes embodied through pathologisation and disavowal. In this chapter, I work with *Anne-Marie Holloway's* narrative to specifically examine the simultaneity of the psychic and social dimensions of abjection. In so doing, I also work with abjection as a simultaneously singular and collective experience. Whereas Deb and Roger focussed on their physical movements between various institutional spaces, Anne-Marie moves figuratively through psychic, social, singular, and collective experiences. Anne-Marie exposes the relationality of abjection: how it moves, and how it is embodied and dispersed psychically and socially, singularly and collectively. Importantly, however, Anne-Marie's narrative also points to the resistance of her own abjection, and I seek to foreground how spaces of possibility can open up for abject bodies to resist their own abjection. In this sense, I am bringing together the arguments made in this book through attention to the narrative of Anne-Marie.

As in Deb and Roger's chapter, I have foregrounded Anne-Marie's own narration of her life. There are multiple ways in which people narrate and account for their lives, yet typically, most have a beginning, middle, and end. Deb and Roger both followed this format. In contrast, Anne-Marie chose to focus her narrative on two moments, and it is these moments that I address in this chapter. What these two moments illuminate is the singular and collective, psychic and social aspects of abjection, and the opportunities in which abjection can be resisted. Anne-Marie's narrative also exposes the fragmentation of her life and her mode of storytelling. I argue that this both reveals the unintelligibility of abject lives and maintains integrity to the ways in which Anne-Marie told her story.

In my first interview with Anne-Marie, the conversation started thus:

> (OK, so if I ask, um, a big broad question, and, can you tell me about
> yourself?)

Mm.

(Take as long as you want)

I'm interested in giving you, um, informa-, information about crime because of the police.

Anne-Marie continued:

When we report things to the police

(Yep)

Like they won't take your calls serious, and they, um, they don't, uh, have any idea how to help people that have got a intellectual disability...

(So why might you call the police?)

Uh, well most people, like, can be scared of domestic violence.

The police arguably constitute a socially abjected group (see Berressem 2007),[1] yet in Anne-Marie's account, they do not know how to engage with her, and proceed to abjectify her. This exposes the degree to which the police, and other abjected groups, can simultaneously be agents or victims of abjection in different temporal and spatial moments. The police in Anne-Marie's narrative are her agents of abjection. In the exchange above it is also interesting how, through use of the collective pronoun 'we', Anne-Marie removes her subject position as a victim of domestic violence and someone labelled 'intellectually disabled'. Who is *we*? Who are these people labelled 'intellectually disabled', or 'victims of domestic violence'? Anne-Marie is talking about victimisation as a collective experience, perhaps as a strategy to mask her (individual) position or to protect herself from her experiences. Is Anne-Marie casting out her own experiences of domestic violence and her subjectivity as someone labelled 'intellectually disabled'? Yet I am also reminded of Butler's (2005: 8) comments that

> the 'I' has no story of its own that is not also the story of a relation—or set of relations—to a set of norms...[and that]...the 'I' is always to some extent dispossessed by the social conditions of its emergence.

In this sense, Anne-Marie's experiences are individual, but they have been socially constituted through a network of relations. In order to resist abjection, then, there has to be a collective set of conditions and agents that make resistance possible. Rather than rely on individuals, a relational ethics is required that resists individual abjection—that which is ultimately collectively created/imposed (see Butler 2004, 2005, 2009).[2]

Anne-Marie chose to focus the bulk of her narrative on her experience with the police. This exchange occurred early in our first interview:

(So you've called the police before?)

Yeah.

(Yep. Can you tell me a little bit more about that?)

Somebody hurt me, and I called the police to escape...

(Support worker: the violence?)

Domestic violence.

(And what did the police do?)

They were rude. They didn't help me. Like I don't exist, like I didn't exist to them...Um, nobody's allowed to hurt, and the police tried to diagnose me, pretty much, when they questioned me. They took my rights away. Uh, I, I, I, they would not let me go, and get help. Yeah...No. No. But the police, they don't help us...They twist things in our head.

(How do they twist things?)

We tell them something different and they're cagey, cagey. Like, they say it didn't happen. And then it's too late to get, a, av-, a-

(Support worker: an, an advocate?)

Yeah, an advocate come in. And then after that it's like our rights have been gone, like, uh, like, we need more support for people to speak for us, in statements, and write down. Because our words are twisted...we're bullied basically by the police.

(So do you think that the police don't trust you?)

They don't know how to treat anybody with an in-, don't know how to treat anybody with an intellectual disability, and they're putting us all in one category. That's where they need the training.

At the start of this exchange, Anne-Marie is talking about her subjective experiences where she is victimised/abjected by her partner, then pathologised/bullied/abjected by the police. Initially she sees the police as her support for her abjection, yet this changes quickly. Anne-Marie describes how the police have treated her as if she does not exist, constituting her as socially dead (Butler 2000, 2015a). Yet she then moves to consider the plight faced by people labelled 'intellectually disabled' more generally.

Anne-Marie moves from *I* and *me*, onwards to *us, our*, and *we*. Cavarero (2000: 90–91) writes: 'The *we* is always positive, the *plural you* is a possible ally, the *they* has the face of an antagonist, the *I* is unseemly, and the [singular] *you* is, of course, superfluous.' Anne-Marie recognises the abjection of disabled lives; it happens to others, not just her. Abjection is a shared, relational, psychic, social, and collective experience. As abjection is shared, resistance must also be shared: the formation of 'bodies in alliance' (Butler 2015b).

The fragmented nature of Anne-Marie's storytelling continued:

(So how did the police treat you?)

They were horrible.

(Horrible? Can you tell me a little bit more information? Or can you tell me a story? Or an example?)

They're not, not allowed to bully me.

(And they bully you?)

Mm. They're not understanding, um, us. At all.

(Can you provide just maybe a little bit more information, or?)

I think, um, people with an intellectual disability, um, are shut down the communication if they don't have the proper support.

(So do you think that the police don't trust your stories, that you say?)

No it's not a matter of trusting, it's when, when we've dropped back, uh, they try to twist things, like we said something but we didn't, didn't. And I think, um, the more we can't, uh, communicate with them, um, well then we get, uh, like anxiety, so they pick up that we're anxious and that, so they try to be sarcastic to us and diagnose us, or whatever, and put us in one category.

(And what category is that?)

Health condition.

(OK. So how much contact have you had with the police?)

It's sorted out, what happened. What happened. But they don't, I don't feel safe ringing them now if something goes wrong…They're meant to help us, but they don't know how to deal with people in the community. See 'cause if you go to the police, they're gonna, they're gonna, um, like, listen to you more because you don't have problem, and I think they judge us that have an intellectual disability. And I suppose if someone else has got a mental, uh, a mental health issue it could be very confuse for the police to work it out. But they're putting people with an intellectual disability all in one category.

In this exchange I have, for a second time, inserted the discourse of trust into our discussion, flagging the possibility that the police may not trust her allegations. This was unintentional at the time, and Anne-Marie rejects it on both occasions. When I raised the possibility on the first occasion she cites ignorance as the factor, and the second time she identifies police manipulation. In any event, Anne-Marie conceives that the issue of trust does not figure in her engagement with the police. Anne-Marie also moves from an individual to a relational, collective experience. She cites communication barriers between herself and the police and then between disabled people and abled people. She is frustrated with the sarcasm, medical diagnosis, and bullying she has received from the police, and she abjects people with 'mental health issue[s]', perhaps in order to protect her own integrity and difference to other abjected bodies. Her abjection has been compounded: first through the violence from her partner and then from the police.

Anne-Marie also brings me—an abled person—into her story, suggesting that I do not have a problem. By doing so, perhaps Anne-Marie conceives disabled subjectivity itself to be a problem or problematic. In any event, in bringing me into the narrative, Anne-Marie is exposing the relationality between us in her account (of abjection). Drawing on the work of Cavarero (2000), Butler (2005: 32) writes that 'one can tell an autobiography only to an other, and one can reference an "I" only in relation to a "you": without the "you," my own story becomes impossible'. In this interlocutory setting, Anne-Marie is highlighting our fundamental sociality and interdependence. Given our shared relationality and dependency, each of us requires an ally to fight and resist our abjection.

My queerness is perhaps unintelligible to Anne-Marie. In conceiving me as not having a 'problem', she does not consider/address my identification with a queer, abjected subjectivity (which I did not disclose to her but that some see written on my body). We can then see how abjection can be invisibilised, not readily recognisable, or not abject at all depending on temporal and spatial contexts and the agents involved. Is there a continuum of abject lives? Given that abject bodies abjectify other abject bodies, it appears there may be. This reminds me again of Baynton's (2001) argument that other socially abjected groups have tried to resist the depiction that they are disabled, thus abjectifying disability as an intolerable social identity. Young (1990) also suggests that queer, disabled, and old bodies are more prone to oppression and discrimination because of their permeability; anyone can become queer, disabled, or old (unlike, arguably, someone becoming 'black', for example). This creates 'border anxiety' (Young 1990: 146), where people must defend their own identity because they are threatened:

> I cannot deny that the old person will be myself, but that means my death, so I avert my gaze from the old person, or treat her as a child, and want to leave her presence as soon as possible.
>
> (Young 1990: 147)

People must abjectify others to preserve their own identity and bodily integrity (Kristeva 1982). In any case, Anne-Marie has been abjected by the police and no longer feels safe in their presence. That Anne-Marie does not feel confident in engaging with the police for support highlights her heightened marginalisation in society. Her own home is not safe, and neither is a police station.

At this point during our first interview, I felt that Anne-Marie was getting increasingly frustrated when she spoke about the police. In hindsight I am not sure whether this was true, but at that stage I was not yet familiar with Anne-Marie's mode of storytelling and her short answers. I decided to change the topic and focus on more background and contextual questions (after all, I mainly used the first interviews as opportunities for rapport-building). I learned that Anne-Marie is 43 years old, she went to boarding school when she was younger, and she struggled with her reading and writing. She has one sister and two brothers, and her biological parents have separated, but they now have new partners. She was born in another large metropolitan city, but she now lives in Sydney because her mum lives in another nearby town.

Anne-Marie must use the train to visit her mum:

(And how do you go catching the train?)

Mm, well sometimes I have difficult.

(What do you have difficulty with?)

Mm, to uh, sometimes I have difficult [three second pause], so I ask people to help me sometimes.

(And do they help you?)

Sometimes they do and sometimes they don't.

(Why do you think some people don't help?)

Because the train master gets busy, that's probably why.

(So you ask the people that work there, do you?)

Yeah…And if they've had a bad day, uh, they take it out on us. Sometimes.

Anne-Marie is speculating as to the reasons why she sometimes does not receive help and is abjected; she may be trying to construct a story that eschews blame. Additionally, Anne-Marie moves from individual to collective experience again; it may be that Anne-Marie finds it more comfortable to talk about collective experiences of maltreatment rather than her individual subjective experiences.

In our second interview the topic returned to the police. Here is the start of the discussion:

(Can you tell me how you first came in contact with the police?)

(Support worker: Why did the police get involved?)

The door, the door…He threw me through the front door, a glass door.

(Threw you through the glass door)

Yeah.

(OK, and did you get hurt? Did you have cuts or anything?)

Yeah.

(Yeah, and so what happened after that?)

The police told me I was crazy.

Anne-Marie was in an abusive relationship with her partner who she lived with for about nine months. One day her partner threw her through a glass door, leaving her with severe mouth injuries. After this,

> Yeah, yeah, yeah. I went to, I went. The people. I ring up on the phone. I ring up the people on the phone, and then they found me, uh, a place, a house. Not my own place, but a refuge here, a refuge. And I went. And then I went to the refuge. Here. I ring up, and the people transferred me to the refuge. Then after that, I went out. Walking. I went walking. Walking. Walking. And then my friend said, um, walking. And then I saw my friend, talking to my friend, and I had a cup of tea with her. My friend, uh, I went walking, I saw my friend walking, I stopped, then we had a coffee in the shop, went in the shop. And she ordered me a drink, and we drink it, a cup of coffee with my friend. And talking. And then, um, my friend noticed, my friend noticed, when I put up the drink, the drink to my mouth, that my, my mouth there was swollen, and I said it was nothing. Then I feel that there was no tooth there.

(And then, so, then you went to the…)

No, she asked me how I lost my tooth, and I didn't know, and then I had a look at the refuge in the mirror, and there was a tooth missing. And then, um, I thought it was nothing. And then, then that night, uh, I, fall, feeling sick and I vomit, and a tooth come out, from there. Out the front it fell out. And then, so, then I went to the, uh, doctor. And talked to the doctor, and asked was I, telling that I had a tooth, the tooth hurt, and it went missing, and I said, asked him about germs and that, in there. And, uh, he said, um, he said, what he said, uh, he said there something there, and yeah, a couple of thing-, and tested it, and another tooth come out when I was in the doctor's surgery, there. So then I went to get it x-rayed, 'cause he referred me to the dental hospital, and 'cause you have to wait, he said it would be urgent for me to get it looked at. So then they sent me there, and then they gave me, uh, ah, x-rays and that. And then they told me to go back to my GP to get a blood test done, to find out if it's calcium, to ask. Or to ask my parents was it gingivitis. But they found there was no gingivitis, so they want to, uh, a test done, a calcium. And then a couple of months after I had the test done for the doctor, the calcium, there was nothing wrong so they, four days later I went to the police. Then they told me I'm crazy. Back here, they tell me I'm crazy. Tried to bully me, or they didn't take me serious.

The events surrounding this are unclear and fragmented, and it is uncertain how much time transpired between the incident with her ex-partner and her contact with the doctor.

On one occasion Anne-Marie said that she went to the doctors two days after being thrown through the door, yet the doctors speculated it was either gingivitis or calcium problems that caused the missing teeth. How could they think this? Would they not have seen the fresh wounds? It is also curious that Anne-Marie only identified her partner as the source of her injuries *after* ruling out germs, gingivitis, or calcium issues. How could she not locate the injuries she sustained? It appears that there is complicity between Anne-Marie and the doctors to hide something. If they addressed the issue, they would have to stop abjecting Anne-Marie, yet there is too much invested in silencing and concealing what has occurred to her. In Anne-Marie's account, her abjection must be invisibilised by herself and the medical staff.

However, it may also be the case that Anne-Marie can only negotiate her abjection with one thing at a time. For example, Anne-Marie has just left her partner and entered (another) abject zone of the refuge (McClintock 1995). Anne-Marie may need to grapple with or make sense of this first, before she chooses, or is forced, to deal with other matters. In any event, Anne-Marie's mouth transforms into an abject object when she must confront what happened to her.

Anne-Marie was asked why she did not go to the police straight away, and she whispered the following answers:

It wasn't a big issue at the time.

(OK. So you just thought that it was, um, normal? Or, how did you look at it?)

Um, yeah. Back here, um, back here. Back here, in here, hold, in pictures, back here. Um, here.

Anne-Marie then pointed at a stock image of a woman looking sad (this picture was in the easy-read information sheet used for the consent process). The conversation continued:

(Take your time, it's alright)

Back here, here, I felt, I felt, back here, I felt sad. And then I didn't think anybody would care.

Anne-Marie felt abject sadness following the event, and she did not know what to do. To me, it felt as if she was ashamed of what happened, and her whispering may support this. Shame, according to Sedgwick and Frank (1995: 133), is 'the effect of indignity, of defeat, of transgression, and of alienation … [it] is felt as an inner torment, a sickness of the soul'. Shame is externally oriented; Anne-Marie is worried what people, including myself, will think of her. This mirrors Deb's fears; disclosing abjection will compound it and constitute her as more abject. Anne-Marie also says she thinks others will not care; she knows how disabled people get treated, and she has trepidations about speaking out.

Anne-Marie stayed at the refuge for a couple of months. At some point she went to the police station to report the domestic violence. She was asked about the event:

(OK, and can you tell me about what happened when you went to the police station?)

Bad thing happened, bad.

(Did the police touch you?)

Bullied me.

(They bullied you. How did they bully you?)

They told me that I, um, that I, that I done it to myself.

(To your teeth?)

Yeah.

(And how did they say that?)

Uh, they tried to then diagnose me, straight away.

After Anne-Marie excluded calcium/gingivitis as the problems that caused the missing teeth, it is unclear how she then concluded it must have been from the violent incident with her partner. Her forgetting and remembering may be a strategic manoeuvre. She may be looking for any other explanation available to her, yet she must confront reality when those theories evaporate.

Incoherence characterises her story. From the interviews I have conducted throughout this research, it appears that abject lives are frequently told in fragmentary and chaotic ways. Is this deliberate? One strategy of abjection might be to make your life, and your narration of that life, incoherent or incomprehensible to others. The violence inflicted upon disabled/abject bodies is incomprehensible to them; they cannot make sense of it, so their justifications and explanations are likewise incomprehensible. Yet there is also a sense in which giving an account of oneself is inherently problematic:

> [i]f I try to give an account of myself, if I try to make myself recognizable and understandable, then I might begin with a narrative account of my life. But this narrative will be disoriented by what is not mine, or not mine alone. And I will, to some degree, have to make myself substitutable in order to make myself recognizable. The narrative authority of the 'I' must give way to the perspective and temporality of a set of norms that contest the singularity of my story.
>
> (Butler 2005: 37)

Any account of oneself is shaped by convention, convenience, discourse, and memory. What Anne-Marie's story does reveal, however, is her resistance to her own abjection. Her partner has assaulted her, and going to the police marks another step (after leaving him) to resist this form of abjection. Yet while she enters the abject zone of a police station, her abjection is compounded when they bully/abjectify her.

The conversation returned to her first encounter with the police:

> the police were rude, that's all.
>
> (And how were they rude?)
>
> Well like, it's like I, um, it's like I've hurt myself to get their attention.
>
> (Is that what they think?)
>
> Yeah.
>
> (And how does that make you feel?)
>
> Well I, then I didn't have any faith in the police. And then, um, then I ignored it, then I went back a couple of months ago, uh, 'cause I saw him, and I got scared.

It is unclear how the police concluded that Anne-Marie's injuries were self-inflicted, and her story points to the communication barriers all too common between disabled and abled people, including the police (Ellem et al. 2008; Goodley 2000; Victorian Equal Opportunity and Human Rights Commission 2014). As Anne-Marie recounts it, the police told her to go away, so she left. Sometime after her first contact with the police, she thinks she saw her (by now) ex-partner in a park. Feeling that he may be following her, Anne-Marie returned to the police station for a second time. If he was following her, by seeking out the assistance of the police a second time, Anne-Marie is trying to resist her perceived abjection.

On her second visit to the police, Anne-Marie said,

> They couldn't do anything, 'cause it was imagination in my head.
>
> (And did they know that you had been there before, and that you told them...)

Yeah 'cause they wrote a statement, but they kept arguing with me the whole time.

(How did they argue?)

Telling me, telling me that I didn't have no rights, like, aggressive, that I had no rights to, to complain to them. I had no rights to complain to them, no rights.

(And how did that make you feel?)

So I didn't do nothing about it.

As disabled people are constantly infantilised (see Luborsky 1994; Robey, Beckley, and Kirschner 2006), and because children are constantly charged with inflating or inventing stories (see Gervais et al. 2000), I argue that this creates an environment in which disabled people, and particularly those labelled 'intellectually disabled', are constituted as unreliable, untrustworthy, indecisive, and prone to confabulation and acquiescence (Slater 2015). That Anne-Marie was not believed, and deemed 'trouble', attests to this point. Anne-Marie left the police station again with no help. She is trying to resist her abjection, to fight back, yet the agents and structures within the police station will not allow her. Just as others are complicit in the constitution of subjects as abject, so it may be the case that abjection cannot be resisted without the complicity of others. In light of the multi-dimensional forms abjection takes and the complicity of others as agents of abjection, it is especially hard for individuals to fight abjection on, and as, their own.

At some point after her second encounter with the police, Anne-Marie contacted a domestic violence service to seek some help. This is another example of Anne-Marie's resistance; one avenue did not work, so she is deploying another strategy to fight back. She understands that she has been treated wrongly, and she is seeking reparation for her abjection. Those at the domestic violence service told Anne-Marie to go back to the police station because she needed to ensure they had statements on the record. On her third visit, the situation escalated:

I went back, and then they locked me up in the cell, telling me I'm crazy. Put me in the cell, and told me to stay there.

(Support worker: so…)

I'm crazy, that's what they said.

(So how did they lock you up in the cell?)

With the keys.

(So, can you try to just, describe it to me in a little bit more detail?)

They put me, you know, the cell in gaol…

(That's silly. Were you being, violent, were you doing anything?)

No, trying to talk to them…'Cause they didn't understand what I was trying to say, but they didn't then get a liaison officer or anyone to help me, or they couldn't be bothered.

The law requires that Anne-Marie should have been assisted by a support worker in her engagement with the police, but evidently this was not the case.[3] It was difficult to ascertain how the police reacted in the way that Anne-Marie described. Like Roger, Anne-Marie spoke with such emotion that it was difficult to ascertain important details in the events she was describing. According to Anne-Marie's account, the police think everything she does is self-inflicted. How are the police able to draw these conclusions? Did they think Anne-Marie was just a troublemaker? Could they not understand her? Was she being threatening or violent? We do not know.

Anne-Marie told me that she was confined to an abject zone (a cell) within an abject zone (police station) for a day, and upon her release,

they gave me fines to pay.

(What were the fines for?)

Public nuisance they said.

On another occasion Anne-Marie added the fines were for:

damaging myself.

(For damaging yourself?)

Yeah, 'cause they're saying I've done that to annoy them.

(So you got charged for hurting yourself?)

Yeah. Because what they're trying to say is I've had a mental illness, not understanding, and they're diagnose me.

(Support worker: And that you made it all up?)

Yeah, what they're saying is I've made allegations to them, and it's not the truth, and they couldn't be bothered. Or they were saying I had delusions when I came and tried to tell them.

Asked how much the fines were, Anne-Marie replied:

they tried to charge me seven thousand dollars, seven thousand dollars' worth, seven thousand!

It is unclear what the fines were for, but speculatively, for public nuisance and making a false report to the police. Anne-Marie was accused of self-abjection, and it is unclear how the situation escalated to such an extent that she was first locked up and, secondly, fined. Anne-Marie also highlights how the police have conflated 'intellectual disability' with 'mental illness', something common in broader (policing) literature (see Hall and Kearns 2001; Office of Police Integrity 2005). According to Anne-Marie's narrative, the police had little idea how to communicate with her. It is also interesting that if the police presumed that Anne-Marie was 'mentally ill', and that that was influencing her behaviour, then how could they fine her? If she was lying because she was mentally ill, then surely the police could not simply issue a fine without acting on their diagnosis of a mental health issue.

But Anne-Marie's resistance is not over. After the police released her, Anne-Marie contacted a disability service for more help. Anne-Marie knows she is being abjected, and her three encounters with the police testify to her continual resistance. Resistance is not a solitary moment; there are different moments at different times that provide opportunities to resist one's situation. For Anne-Marie, communication barriers made it difficult:

Yeah. It took a long while to sort it out, with them, too.

(Mhm)

To find out what exactly did happen, 'cause they couldn't get any sense out of it [laughter from Anne-Marie].

I can recognise how the police officers may have struggled to understand Anne-Marie. It took three interviews with her until I gathered a semi-coherent narrative of what had occurred. She spoke in short bursts, lots of emotion, and often ignored questions. However, rather than blaming Anne-Marie and other disabled people for their 'poor communicative abilities', I hold ableist society accountable for the ways in which disabled people are constituted as having poor communication skills. It is abled people who need to change, not disabled people. Bartkowiak-Théron, Asquith, and Roberts (2017) argue that the police need to develop deeper cultural capability in order to appreciate the differences between people with multiple and intersecting vulnerabilities. This is especially important when police and other criminal justice agents are sometimes found to be *more* combative or confrontational towards populations they do not understand or are unfamiliar with (see Dwyer 2014; Henshaw and Thomas 2012), and this is also evidenced in Anne-Marie's narrative. Instead of focussing on how disabled people should speak *normally*, there needs to be a refocus on the *normality of disabled people speaking differently*, and an appreciation of the cultural capabilities required to understand those differences (Hansen and Philo 2007).

With the help of the disability service, Anne-Marie went to the state's Anti-Discrimination Board about her encounters with the police. She explains the outcome:

the Minister of Police did have a meeting with us and said, uh, talked to us and said they were sorry how I was treated and that, and then they said I didn't have any fines and that. But, still didn't help me, the damage was done. Because when I went to the domestic violence liaison officer I couldn't charge him for my teeth 'cause it was so long ago.

As Anne-Marie describes at the end of this passage, the violence/abjection from her ex-partner that led to her engagement with the police has still not been properly investigated. As evidenced by broader literature (see Sin 2013; Sin et al. 2009), there is too much focus on dealing with and diagnosing disabled people than actually addressing their real-world concerns. What message does this send to Anne-Marie? That her abjection does not matter? The effect of not investigating compounds her abjection and works to ontologically invalidate her and her experiences (Campbell 2015; Hughes 2012).

Once Anne-Marie had told me about her encounters with the police, I asked her to reflect:

(So do you think that if, God forbid, if something happened to you in the next, let's say week, where something bad happened to you, would you feel confident going to the police?)

No.

(So what would you do?)

Nothing.

(Is that scary?)

I don't know, we have to live with it. Because that's how people with intellectual disability get treated.

(Mhm)

Unless I had proper support, that somebody would help me. But it depends, you know.

This is perhaps unsurprising; Anne-Marie's response to abjection is to do nothing, because her last attempts did not result in any form of productive outcome regarding her experience of domestic violence, and in fact made her position worse.

It appears in this section of the narrative that Anne-Marie is resigned to her own abjection. Anne-Marie also moves again from an individual to collective experience. She understands that it is a collective set of experiences that people labelled 'intellectually disabled' face on a broader, often daily basis. Yet she has not given up completely; she flags that she needs greater support, and this again points towards her resistance to her own abjection, and the acknowledgement that resistance requires a collective and relational— rather than individual—set of circumstances and practices.

Anne-Marie added,

> That's why a lot of women won't go to the police, when they're in a domestic violence, that do have an intellectual disability. We're blocking ourselves not going there.

Anne-Marie looks inwardly at disabled bodies, yet I suggest this gaze is more useful when turned outward to the ways in which ableist and disablist discourses constitute disabled people. In an environment where there are a collective set of experiences inflicted upon disabled bodies, the response requires a collective set of responses from multiple agents over time and space. I asked Anne-Marie if she thought people labelled 'intellectually disabled' get treated worse by the police, and she replied:

> Yeah, 'cause if you went to court they'd treat you differently from what you've done, then me, they look at me differently.

(And how...)

> More judgmental towards us.

Again, Anne-Marie moves from the individual to collective, and she constitutes me as non-abject (or perhaps, less abject). Anne-Marie is aware of her social position, and recognises she is treated worse than others. She also knows that this is unfair, and she has tried to resist the depiction that she is *less than*, or that her abjection does not matter.

Due to Anne-Marie's (chaotic) mode of storytelling, I decided to focus on one incident at a time before moving to different topics that she had previously introduced. Once a more complete picture of the police incident arose (over the course of three interviews), I then turned to the experience with her ex-partner and the nature of their relationship. Anne-Marie said,

> I was living with this person for nine, for nine months. And he punched me, and then I felt that it was OK. I couldn't build confidence, but then I was getting bruises and people were questioning me.

Anne-Marie's abjection has been distributed throughout parts of her body (bruises). Her normalisation of violence also mirrors many women's accounts of intimate-partner violence (see Edwards, Dardis, and Gidycz 2011; Pestka and Wendt 2014). Anne-Marie understands how people labelled 'intellectually disabled' are treated by society, such that when she is abjected herself she perceives it as 'normal'. Anne-Marie continued:

And then my friend say 'Oh, what happened?' 'I fell over, I fell over'. She said 'Oh, you better go to the doctor'. Because my friend was, uh, concerned. 'Cause I had an intellectual disability that I had no balance, and she wanted to come to the doctor. And then I said 'Oh, it'll get better, don't worry'. And when my shoulder was bruised, she saw me again holding my shoulder, 'What happened?' 'Nothing I fell again'. And she said 'Oh, uh, my friend told me, um, uh, you need to go to the doctor because she said, uh, some people can fall and it could be a balance problem'.

Like the incident with the teeth, Anne-Marie must construct a story that invisibilises her own abjection. Anne-Marie continued:

And then I con-, and then I didn't want to contact my friend anymore, because then here, back here, back here in the pictures here, here, in here, this one. [Starts whispering] I didn't want to tell my friend, I didn't want to tell my friend that I was sad.

Anne-Marie pointed to the same image she did earlier. Anne-Marie recognises her predicament, and she is trying to hide it from her friends. The consequences of her abjection do not start and stop at physical violence; it has moved to Anne-Marie isolating herself from her friends. Abjection spreads, and creates loneliness.

I asked Anne-Marie more about her ex-partner:

(So, do you think you can tell me a little bit about [your ex-partner]?)

He's crazy…Yeah well he's got a mental illness, but it's against his religion to take medication…

(…how did you meet [your ex-partner]?)

Through friends.

(Through friends. And was he nice to you at the start?)

Kind of.

(Yep. And so then you, you started seeing him?)

No I moved in with him.

(You moved in with him, OK)

Mhm.

(And he didn't treat you very nice?)

No…Yeah he's got, he's got, uh, bipolar he said.

(OK. And so, why do you think he was not treating you very nice?)

I don't know [pause]. I suppose he, people have split personality with bipolar as well, I don't know.

Like the police officers who diagnosed her, Anne-Marie is now diagnosing her ex-partner as crazy, mentally ill, split personality, and bipolar. She is disavowing the violence inflicted upon her, and abjecting her ex-partner. Why does Anne-Marie do this? She knows that when the police diagnosed her, they locked her in a cell and fined her. Yet it may be that because Anne-Marie knows that violence was inflicted upon her when she was diagnosed/abjected, she may be able to do the same to her partner (that is, diagnose and then punish him).

The conversation digressed on to other matters, but we later returned:

(So, if we can take one step back, and talk about [your ex-partner] a little bit more. And so he treated you badly?)

Mm [nods].

(Was this, um, so he was verbally abusive, so he said nasty things to you?)

Mm.

(Is that true, or not?)

Mm, yeah [nods].

(And so what kind of things would he say?)

I don't remember now, it's so long ago.

(OK. And so he was also physically abusive?)

Yeah and that's when I tried to put boundaries in place, and got hurt.

At another point, Anne-Marie added,

And then here, I didn't, I was talking to him and trying to tell him to stop, and he, and that's when he yelled at me, more. I was trying to tell him to stop.

Here Anne-Marie has tried to put boundaries in place between herself and her ex-partner, and this is reminiscent of Deb's approaches with her sexual violators and her ex-partner, David. Deb was perhaps better able to negotiate these transactions because in Anne-Marie's account, the instantiation of boundaries intensified her abjection. When abject bodies try to resist their abjection, a sense of disruption occurs for the non-abject, such that they try to put the abject back in their place. The non-abject cannot deal with the destabilisation of dis/ability, abjection, and ab/normality. What Deb and Anne-Marie's stories do illuminate, however, is that abjection can only be resisted with the support of external structures and allies within favourable temporal and spatial moments. Collectively there are possibilities, yet individually the opportunities are potentially more restricted.

Towards the end of our conversations about her ex-partner, the following exchange took place:

> He hit me, and then I tried to put boundaries in place, and that's when he threw me through the front door, and I don't know why, if it's the way I've come across towards how it's been said.
>
> (What do you mean by that, sorry? [Pause] Do you mean if, um, if he took what you said the wrong way…)
>
> No you say 'Stop!' You tell someone to stop and put boundaries in place.
>
> (Yep)
>
> But I think it's what people want to hear, how they deal with it, and it's how he deals with it, went through the front door.
>
> (OK. And so I'll just ask you one more time…)
>
> Mm
>
> (…but just think about it, you know, for as long as you like, but do you know why he was doing this to you? [Six second pause] Because obviously he was being terrible)
>
> Maybe he was drinking when he was working during the day, but I don't know.

Like Anne-Marie's previous stories, she may be trying to find other explanations because she does not want to confront or engage with her partner's violence. She may be blaming herself, which is an act of self-abjection. Anne-Marie's comments above marked our last conversation on the topic.

By the time a semi-coherent account of the police incident and her relationship with her ex-partner was covered, there was not much time to discuss other aspects of Anne-Marie's life. However, it seemed that Anne-Marie only wanted to talk about those two topics. This was very similar to the interviews I conducted with *Warren Goodwin, Richard Brady,* and *Emma Silva.* Warren only wanted to talk about his experience of sexual assault and being gay, Richard did not want to talk about his experiences in the asylum, and Emma only wanted to discuss her difficulties seeking employment and other bureaucratic issues. This did not concern me as I was only interested in what each participant chose to tell me. Anne-Marie did want to talk about disability generally, and she told me she sometimes does not disclose her disabled subjectivity to others, because sometimes people misinterpret what an intellectual disability is.

Perhaps Anne-Marie's experiences with the police have figured into her decision-making. For Anne-Marie, it may be that identifying as disabled brings greater risk.

In our third interview we spoke more about disability:

(So, do you identify as someone with a disability?)

Yes.

(Yep, and so what does that mean to you?)

It means that we're challenged more than other people.

I was not able to ascertain in what ways disabled people are challenged more, but again Anne-Marie moves from the individual to the collective. It may be that Anne-Marie is more guarded about her disabled subjectivity because of the abjection is has brought her from the police. Further, she had little sense that anything could be done about it:

Well you can't change people's attitudes, that's human nature...It could just be their attitude, how they speak to you.

(Mhm. And how do some people speak to you?)

It depends, if people are having a bad day they may take it out on people, and then it could just be their, their nature...And people with intellectual disability shouldn't take that personally, with bad attitude.

In this exchange it appears that Anne-Marie may think that all people can be treated poorly and indiscriminately, and that disabled people are not targeted/abjected in particular. Yet her earlier comments suggest she recognises the abjection of disabled lives. Perhaps this is another example of Anne-Marie seeking to avoid apportioning blame, and absolving others of their bad attitudes towards disabled people.

Anne-Marie did not choose to reveal much else to me. When asked to describe her personality, Anne-Marie said,

I'm outgoing and then sometimes I draw back.

I also asked her,

(So, what matters the most to you, do you think?)

It's not to be judged.

Anne-Marie knows the treatment she and other disabled people receive, she knows it is wrong, and in her account she has resisted her abjection and illustrated her desire to be non-abject. Yet her story also points to the ways in which resistance must be collectively and relationally facilitated. We cannot leave it up to individuals to take responsibility for their own abjection when there a collective set of conditions that abjectify disabled bodies in the first instance.

Considering Anne-Marie's story

In Anne-Marie's life history narrative, two incidents stand out: the violence from her partner and the violence from the police. In each of these encounters, Anne-Marie has resisted her abjection. She left her partner, and she got an apology from the police. Many responses are available in the face of abjection: transforming it (Genet 1966 [1951]), finding unexpected opportunity (Halperin 2007), conceiving it a dirty secret (Warner 1995), and resignifying the symbolic domain (Butler 1993). Is Anne-Marie's resistance what Butler (1993; in Meijer and Prins 1998), Halperin (2007), Warner (1995), and Genet (1966 [1951]) had in mind? I think so; each attempts, in differing ways, to disarm or resist abjection, and Anne-Marie's narrative demonstrates how resistance to abjection takes many forms and is mobilised in different temporal and spatial moments.

Resistance requires the cooperation of agents who act with each other whenever and wherever it feels possible, and for whatever reason. I am reminded of Halperin's (2007: 84) reflection on Genet's story that 'some people ... might simply be crushed'. Anne-Marie's story demonstrates this; she was repeatedly crushed by her partner until circumstances enabled her to resist, and she was repeatedly crushed by the police until another set of circumstances allowed reparation. I suggest that resistance—like abjection— is not singular and, thus, is in social circulation to be taken up when practicable. We have seen, in each of the preceding chapters, how the participants in this research have variously sought to resist their abjection in small ways and in small moments. Resistance *can be* a response to social abjection, yet ultimately, a relational ethics is required in order for this to flourish. In the next and final chapter, I turn to this question of possibilities for resistance and for imagining disability otherwise.

Notes

1 This is under-theorised in abject literature, yet police officers are considered legitimate categories of hate crime victims in some jurisdictions, and this signifies their oppression in certain temporal/spatial contexts (Grattet and Jenness 2001).
2 I also turn to this point in Chapter 8.
3 Yet it should also be highlighted that the date of this incident is unclear. If it occurred prior to 2005 such a requirement would not have been in place. At the time of the interviews in 2015, Anne-Marie said the incident happened 'two years ago or more', indicating that it happened most likely after 2005.

References

Bartkowiak-Théron, I, Asquith, NL, and Roberts, KA 2017, 'Vulnerability as a Contemporary Challenge for Policing', in *Policing Encounters with Vulnerability*, edited by NL Asquith, I Bartkowiak-Théron, and KA Roberts, Palgrave Macmillan, London, pp. 1–23.

Baynton, DC 2001, 'Disability and the Justification of Inequality in American History', in *The New Disability History: American Perspectives*, edited by PK Longmore and L Umansky, New York University Press, New York and London, pp. 33–57.

Berressem, H 2007, 'On the Matter of Abjection', in *The Abject of Desire: The Aestheticization of the Unaesthetic in Contemporary Literature and Culture*, edited by K Kutzbach and M Mueller, Rodopi, Amsterdam and New York, pp. 19–48.

Butler, J 1993, *Bodies that Matter: On the Discursive Limits of 'Sex'*, Routledge, New York and London.

Butler, J 2000, *Antigone's Claim: Kinship between Life and Death*, Columbia University Press, New York.

Butler, J 2004, *Precarious Life: The Powers of Mourning and Violence*, Verso, London and New York.

Butler, J 2005, *Giving an Account of Oneself*, Fordham University Press, New York.

Butler, J 2009, *Frames of War: When Is Life Grievable?* Verso, London and New York.

Butler, J 2015b, *Notes toward a Performative Theory of Assembly*, Harvard University Press, Cambridge, MA.

Butler, J 2015a, *Senses of the Subject*, Fordham University Press, New York.

Campbell, FK 2015, 'Legislating Disability: Negative Ontologies and the Government of Legal Identities', in *Foucault and the Government of Disability*, 2nd edition, edited by S Tremain, University of Michigan Press, Ann Arbor, MI, pp. 108–130.

Cavarero, A 2000, *Relating Narratives: Storytelling and Selfhood*, translated by PA Kottman, Routledge, London and New York, [originally published as *Tu che mi guardi, tu che mi racconti*, Giagiacomo Feltrinelli, Milan, 1997].

Dwyer, A 2014, '"We're Not like These Weird Feather Boa-Covered AIDS-Spreading Monsters": How LGBT Young People and Service Providers Think Riskiness Informs LGBT Youth-Police Interactions', *Critical Criminology*, 22(1): 65–79.

Edwards, KM, Dardis, CM, and Gidycz, CA 2011, 'Women's Disclosure of Dating Violence: A Mixed Methodological Study', *Feminism & Psychology*, 22(4): 507–517.

Ellem, K, Wilson, J, Chui, WH, and Knox, M 2008, 'Ethical Challenges of Life Story Research with Ex-Prisoners with Intellectual Disability', *Disability & Society*, 23(5): 497–509.

Genet, J 1966, *Miracle of the Rose*, Grove Press, New York, translated by Bernard Frechtman, [originally published as *Miracle de la rose*, Librairie Gallimard, 1951].

Gervais, J, Tremblay, RE, Desmarais-Gervais, L, and Vitaro, F 2000, 'Children's Persistent Lying, Gender Difference, and Disruptive Behaviours: A Longitudinal Perspective', *International Journal of Behavioral Development*, 24(2): 213–221.

Goodley, D 2000, *Self-Advocacy in the Lives of People with Learning Difficulties: The Politics of Resilience*, Open University Press, Buckingham and Philadelphia, PA.

Grattet, R and Jenness, V 2001, 'Examining the Boundaries of Hate Crime Law: Disabilities and the "Dilemma of Difference"', *The Journal of Criminal Law & Criminology*, 91(3): 653–698.

Hall, E and Kearns, R 2001, 'Making Space for the "Intellectual" in Geographies of Disability', *Health & Place*, 7(3): 237–246.

Halperin, DM 2007, *What Do Gay Men Want? An Essay on Sex, Risk, and Subjectivity*, The University of Michigan Press, Ann Arbor, MI.

Hansen, N and Philo, C 2007, "The Normality of Doing Things Differently: Bodies, Spaces and Disability Geography', *Tijdschrift voor Economische en Sociale Geografie*, 98(4): 493–506.

Henshaw, M and Thomas, S 2012, 'Police Encounters with People with Intellectual Disability: Prevalence, Characteristics and Challenges', *Journal of Intellectual Disability Research*, 56(6): 620–631.

Hughes, B 2012, 'Civilising Modernity and the Ontological Invalidation of Disabled People', in *Disability and Social Theory: New Developments and Directions*, edited by D Goodley, B Hughes, and L Davis, Palgrave Macmillan, London, pp. 17–32.

Kristeva, J 1982, *Powers of Horror: An Essay on Abjection*, translated by LS Roudiez, Columbia University Press, New York.

Luborsky, MR 1994, 'The Cultural Adversity of Physical Disability: Erosion of Full Adult Personhood', *Journal of Aging Studies*, 8(3): 239–253.

McClintock, A 1995, *Imperial Leather: Race, Gender and Sexuality in the Colonial Contest*, Routledge, New York and London.

Meijer, IC and Prins, B (with J Butler) 1998, 'How Bodies Come to Matter: An Interview with Judith Butler', *Signs: Journal of Women in Culture and Society*, 23(2): 275–286.

Office of Police Integrity 2005, *Review of Fatal Shootings by Victoria Police*, Office of Police Integrity, Victorian Government Printer, Melbourne.

Pestka, K and Wendt, S 2014, 'Belonging: Women Living with Intellectual Disabilities and Experiences of Domestic Violence', *Disability & Society*, 29(7): 1031–1045.

Robey, KL, Beckley, L, and Kirschner, M 2006, 'Implicit Infantilizing Attitudes about Disability', *Journal of Developmental and Physical Disabilities*, 18(4): 441–453.

Sedgwick, EK and Frank, A 1995, 'Shame-Humiliation and Contempt-Disgust', in *Shame and Its Sisters: A Silvan Tomkins Reader*, edited by EK Sedgwick and A Frank, Duke University Press, Durham, NC and London, pp. 133–178.

Sin, CH 2013, 'Making Disablist Hate Crime Visible: Addressing the Challenges of Improving Reporting', in *Disability, Hate Crime and Violence*, edited by A Roulstone and H Mason-Bish, Routledge, London and New York, pp. 147–165.

Sin, CH, Hedges, A, Cook, C, Mguni, N, and Comber, N 2009, *Disabled People's Experiences of Targeted Violence and Hostility*, Equality and Human Rights Commission, Research Report 21, Manchester, UK.

Slater, J 2015, *Youth and Disability: A Challenge to Mr Reasonable*, Ashgate Publishing, London.

Victorian Equal Opportunity and Human Rights Commission 2014, *Beyond Doubt: The Experiences of People with Disabilities Reporting Crime—Research Findings*, Victorian Equal Opportunity and Human Rights Commission, Melbourne.

Warner, M 1995, 'Unsafe: Why Gay Men Are Having Risky Sex', *The Village Voice*, January 31, pp. 33–36.

Young, IM 1990, *Justice and the Politics of Difference*, Princeton University Press, Princeton, NJ.

8 Reflections, possibilities, and resistance

Thinking differently about disability and the terms of un/intelligibility has required a new repertoire of terms, concepts, and theories. While summarising my main reflections and arguments in this conclusion, I am cautious about offering any form of conclusive testimony in a book that has inevitably led to more questions than answers. Instead, my aim is to both consolidate and extend my account of abjection. Specifically, in this chapter, I turn to the question of how we respond ethically and politically to the abjection of disabled lives. After offering an account of what I have argued thus far, I move on to consider how this research has heightened my sense of precarity and precariousness. Rather than sideline or disavow these feelings, I engage with them and consider the relation between the participants, me, and you, the reader. Abjection is relational and contagious, and I am moved to consider how we respond to the precarity and precariousness that abjection has created for us. I advocate for resistance, both as a collective and relational practice, and in an effort to resist abjection, provide three inter-related possibilities that shift the gaze from disabled bodies to ableist practices.

What has been (un)learnt?

So what have we learnt? Or, what have we thought to be the case, only to find that it is not? At the outset of this book, I proposed that I was intent on examining abjection as a lived social practice. In and through thirteen life histories I have explored the social and psychic, individual and collective dimensions of abjection.

In 'Beginnings', I traced how I arrived at this research topic, and I introduced the epistemological standpoints I have taken in this research. Essentialist understandings of disability were problematised and disrupted in order to illustrate how disability is discursively constructed. Additionally, the frame of 'violence' was identified as too restrictive in analysing the participants' accounts, and that the theory of the abject better accounted for the oppression of disabled people. The theory of the abject was introduced, first, through the lens of Kristeva's (1982) psychoanalytic account, and then complemented with McClintock's (1995) seven dimensions of abjection.

Through this conceptualisation, the aims of the research were introduced, and I illustrated how abjection was to be interrogated as a psychic and social, individual and collective experience. Importantly, however, I also documented my emphasis in exploring the spaces of possibility in which abjection can be resisted.

In 'Social Abjection and Reappropriation', I extended my account of abjection by addressing Butler's (1993; in Meijer and Prins 1998) theorisations. In addition to Kristeva's (1982) psychoanalytic framing, I introduced Butler's (1993; in Meijer and Prins 1998) conception of abjection as a discursive and political process. Importantly, however, Butler's (1993; in Meijer and Prins 1998) theorisations exposed how abjection could be used to rearticulate the terms of cultural intelligibility, such that abjection can be resisted, reclaimed, and/or reimagined. In order to explore such possibilities against the backdrop of reappropriation, I considered how terms and social practices can be reappropriated through the development/application of crip theory. Abjection itself can be reappropriated, paradoxically, by embracing or reimagining it differently (Halperin 2007). This consideration was important in exposing the spaces of possibility where the terms of cultural intelligibility could be recast.

'Deb's Narrative: Exploring the Multi-Dimensional Forms of Abjection' was the first chapter to introduce the reader to the participants in more detail. In this chapter, Deb and her experiences of abjection were considered using McClintock's (1995) framework and Butler (1993; in Meijer and Prins 1998) and Kristeva's (1982) theorisations. Deb's narrative exposes how abjection is distributed, cyclical, compounding, and often invisible. Deb's story highlights how abjection creates a double bind, through which she is constituted as abject no matter what improvisations she makes. Deb's narrative documents how she was regulated and violated through many of the institutional spaces she passed through and how abjection became a transaction through which she negotiated the world. Deb showed how abjection is shared, contagious, and relational, and how its distribution also limits agency. Her story illustrated the spatial and temporal contours of abjection; that is, where it is used at different moments, at different times, by different people, and with different intensities. Deb's story also showed how abjection can become normalised, but more importantly, how it can also be resisted. While abjection can be cyclical, Deb's story highlights that spaces and possibilities for resistance can emerge from abjection.

Compared to Deb, 'Roger's Narrative: Abjection Amidst Chaos and Fragmentation' highlighted how similar and distinct forms of abjection result in dis/similar outcomes and experiences. Whereas Deb experienced abjection as a cyclical experience, Roger's life history narrative exposed fragmentation, opacity, and uncertainty. Roger's life history narrative also exposed how abjection is a constant threat—even from 'friends'—and that abject bodies are constantly subjected to the authority of others. Importantly, Roger's story also showed how resistance to abjection is difficult. While he now resists through his engagement with disability self-advocacy work, his life has no clear resolution, or 'agential cut' (Barad 2007), such as that in Deb's narrative.

'Eleven Lives' switched registers to introduce and personalise, in more detail, the remaining eleven participants in this research. Part of the purpose of the chapter was to contextualise the chapter that followed, '(Psychic) Self-Abjection: Pathologisation and Disavowal', where I considered how exterior forces of abjection worked their way into the psychic life of many of the participants in this research. Compared to the chapters on Deb and Roger, which largely focussed on the exterior forces of abjection, this chapter focussed on the interiorisation of abjection, and illuminated how the participants drew upon normative discourses of pathology, abnormality, and disavowal in constructing their own disabled subjectivities. This revealed the extent to which the participants in this research embody disablist and ableist norms, and the corporeal imprint of this psychic self-harm.

'Anne-Marie's Narrative: Abjection and Resistance' further teased out the simultaneous relation between the psychic and the social, individual and collective dimensions of abjection through the life history narrative of Anne-Marie. Important in Anne-Marie's narrative was her resistance to the multi-dimensional forms of abjection she encountered. However, Anne-Marie's life history narrative also exposed how resistance sometimes fails, requires perseverance, or demands alliance with others. Consequently, in that chapter, I lay out possibilities for a collective response to abjection, which requires a relational ethics that resists or reclaims abjection. The multi-dimensional forms of abjection encountered by Anne-Marie necessitate a collective response in order to disarm the ability to abject disabled and other precarious bodies.

This research has shown that disabled people are abjected and that multiple forms of abjection conspire at different times and in different moments to *put disabled people in their place*. Abjection works as a social and psychic practice, and regulatory norms work to abjectify and pathologise disabled bodies. But within the thirteen participants' narratives in this research, I have highlighted spaces of possibility where abjection has been resisted. But I ask again: where has this left us?

When I started the project upon which this book is based I set out to study hate crime, yet I have ended up here. Where is *here*, how did I get here, and where will I go next? I have learnt more than I imagined, but I still have questions. What would my participants think of what I have said about them? And how would I articulate to them what I have argued? What would Deb think if I told her that I 'caught' her abjection? What would Warren think if he saw me gag when he ate? How would my participants respond if I told them that they were abject; and what might they say if I told them to resist or reclaim it? Would any of them *claim crip*? And in my unintentional moments of ableism, would they think I am a traitor? Was I never an ally in the first place?

In thinking through this, I am struck by the participants' precarity and precariousness, and I turn to contemplate how abjection is shared. Precarity, for Butler (2015: 33), refers to 'that politically induced condition in which certain populations suffer ... and become differentially exposed to injury, violence and death'. These certain populations include women, queers, transgender people, the poor, disabled people, the stateless, and religious and racial minorities (Butler 2015: 58). Butler (2009, 2015) differentiates between precariousness as a universal condition/vulnerability by virtue of our corporeal embodiment, and precarity as a situational vulnerability that unequally exposes certain populations to the risk of violence and oppression (Mills 2015).

The participants in this research experience precarity and precariousness. They have each told us of different moments throughout their lives that felt unliveable; where death was a real possibility. Clifton was nearly drowned, Roger almost jumped off a bridge, and Peter thought of suicide. Deb was raped, Warren sexually assaulted, and Anne-Marie beaten by her partner. Joshua, Amal, and Jake were bullied at school, and Lisa was bullied in her family. Richard and Freddie have both been bashed, and Emma gets abused on public transport. But these are not solitary or isolated events, and I could have drawn upon many other examples. Violence, as abjection, has been constant, repetitive, and compounding in their lives. They are abject, and this has not only heightened their precarity, but has also highlighted the precariousness of life itself.

Yet I am also struck by my own precarity and precariousness. I was always already abject (perhaps), yet this has intensified in my mind over the past few years. Reflecting on the life histories of the thirteen people in this project, I am also reminded of my own life history, and particularly the precariousness and precarity experienced throughout this research. I am conscious of the ethics and politics of asking people about their experiences of violence/abjection. I am also reminded by Swain, Heyman, and Gillman's (1998) suggestion that research which invites disclosure of experiences of violence can itself be an act of violence. And so, in giving an account of abjection as a collective practice, I feel compelled to expose my own vulnerability, abjection, and precarity. I thus engage in a performative politics that seeks to address collective abjection and the ethics of research.

I cannot reconcile invisibilising my own abjection while foregrounding that of the people who shared their life histories with me, especially as I am trying to confront our collective vulnerability. Let me signpost a few contemplations that arose from the very act of writing this concluding chapter.

> *Research.* How do I access this research population? How do I maintain access? How do I develop rapport? How do I deal with the profound things that they tell me? How do I write well? How do I prioritise my time? How can I understand these theories, and then apply, critique, or shape them?

Yet there were other events in my personal life that occurred throughout the course of this project, and they have taken on new meanings and altered the ways in which I think about them. If I was not studying dis/ability, abjection, violence, subjectivity, and normativity, who knows how I would have constituted them and what significance they might have had?

Deb and Warren. Deb's stories often entered my thoughts, and sometimes my dreams. My interaction with Warren still makes me feel ashamed.

HIV. Why was I self-destructive? Like McRuer (2006: 57), I too engaged in practices where 'HIV was unquestionably on the other side of the condom'. I went even further, abandoning the condom completely. What was I doing? Was my work with abjection seducing me? Was I, as Halperin (2007: 91) proposes, tempting HIV infection 'as a scary but inspired expression of antisocial solidarity with … [my] sick and dead comrades in ignominy'? Or maybe I was just looking for a roadblock between me and a completed project. The prospect of becoming HIV positive offered a justification, albeit extreme, to give up on my work. Maybe abjection became my dirty secret.

Violation. Why did I drink so much? Why did I not scream louder? Or scream out for help? But then I think: it was surely not as bad as the experiences of others? What would I have done differently? How do others feel about their experiences of violation?

Temporary Abledness. What if I become disabled? How would I feel about it? Should I be worried? Am I lying to myself? Am I ableist if I fear becoming disabled? What does that say about me, and my research?

Life and Death. Why am I thinking about death so much lately? Why does my body and mind clench whenever I walk across a street? What if I die before someone reads these words? The recognition of my own bodily vulnerability has intensified in my mind.

Yet I have persevered and resisted. I have shared some details about myself, and have intentionally kept some details vague. My intention is not to be self-indulgent, but merely to highlight how my own abjection, precarity, and precariousness have been produced or exposed and opened to reflection throughout this research.

So I have spoken about the participants and myself, but what about the reader? They will inevitably be precarious (a universal and ontological vulnerability [Butler 2015]), yet will they experience precarity? Will they be disabled or not? Will they occupy another abjected group? Will they be moved by the stories in this text? Will abjection be contagious for them? Will they find my arguments unsettling, compelling, or uncomfortable?

In thinking about the relationality of abjection and precarity, and the relation between the participants, myself, and the reader, the question seems to be: what do we do about this precarity induced by abjection? I start by compelling people to become allies:

> [a]lliances that have formed to exercise the rights of gender and sexual minorities must, in my view, forms links, however difficult, with the diversity of their own population and all the links that implies with other populations subjected to conditions of induced precarity during our time.
>
> (Butler 2015: 67–68)

To enact a politics of this sort, the participants, myself, and the reader need to recognise our interdependency and relatedness to each other. Alliances between all those who experience precarity are equally necessary for a politics of this type. Human lives are relational, interdependent, and co-constitutive, and they cannot live without the support of others (Butler 2015). As Butler (2015: 84, 88) suggests, 'there can be no embodied life without social and institutional support', and 'no human can be human without acting in concert with others'. I propose that a collective and relational response to abjection is therefore necessary. Resistance or reclamation is critical, but cannot be done on one's own. Given the multi-dimensional forms of abjection, any resistance or reclamation can result in being crushed (Halperin 2007). As the participants have shown in this research, fighting back has proven hard and sometimes worsened their situation. Resistance, then, requires the complicity and action of multiple agents.

In articulating possibilities for a relational ethics that resists or reclaims abjection, in this final chapter, I give an account of multiple iterations of resistance drawn from the life histories of the people who participated in this research. First, bearing in mind the moments of resistance in Deb, Roger, and Anne-Marie's narratives, I introduce examples from the narratives of the remaining ten participants to further consider instances in which abjection can be, and *has been*, resisted. Recognising, however, that resistance can be understood as a relational rather than individual practice, I propose a relational, coalitional ethics. I then go on to consider collective possibilities for problematising ableism, disablism, and abjection.

Resisting (individual) abjection

Given the stories in this book, it may appear that abjection is difficult, if not impossible, to resist. However, throughout this book I have opened up a counter-narrative to this argument and foregrounded instances in which the participants in this research have been able to resist their abjection. Before I essay several arguments about how abjection can be resisted as a collective practice, I turn to consider several instances in this research where participants have successfully been able to mount resistance to their abjection. Each of their performances is of different size; some stories of resistance, at first glance, might seem small or inconsequential, yet others may seem drastic. My list is not exhaustive, and I aim merely to expose the different possibilities for resistance available in different spatial and temporal moments for disabled/abject bodies. I then move on to consider how abjection might be more successfully resisted as a collective practice.

(Different) Bodies on public display

Amal is blind and she walks down the street with the aid of a cane. Clifton has cerebral palsy on one side of his body and similarly walks down the street. Warren can only leave the house with a wheelchair, while Lisa and Roger choose to use their wheelchairs occasionally, only when required. Richard has physical differences and he, too, in going about his daily business, walks down the street. Emma, Jake, and Joshua all have their driver's license, and drive when they desire. Each of these people goes about their lives in public. They all look non-normative, and they are, most often, constituted as 'freaks' subjected to the public gaze (Garland Thomson 1997, 2009; Michalko 1999, 2002; Reeve 2002). People look and stare at them. Sometimes people attack them. Some are curious, some disgusted, and some fascinated by them. Some feel pity, and others ignore them:

> [i]t is not only physical limitations that restrict us to our homes and those whom we know. It is the knowledge that each entry into the public world will be dominated by stares, condescension, by pity and by hostility.
>
> (Morris 1991: 25)

In this social world, then, the act of being in public for those who look different is a performative, radical, and resistant act. Clare (2015: 110) calls it flaunting:

> [t]hey are in effect saying to nondisabled people, 'Damn right, you better look. Look long and hard. Watch my crooked hobble, my twitching body, my withered legs. Listen to my hands sign a language you don't even know. Notice my milky eyes I no longer hide behind sunglasses. Look at me straight on, because for all your years of gawking, you've still not seen me.'

In these moments, disabled people are resisting the discourse that disabled people should be living private lives in their homes, out of view from the public (Michalko 2002). Most importantly, however, is that Amal, Clifton, Warren, Lisa, Roger, Richard, Emma, Jake, Joshua, and many other disabled people are confronting abled people about their own corporeality. The presence of disability provokes ontological insecurities in the minds of abled people; confrontations with disabled subjects shatter illusions of invulnerability and expose the abled to their own fragility (Michalko 2002). To be in public, and to show off one's non-normative body, is a performative act of resistance that crips the physical environment, and foregrounds the fragmentary, permeable, and 'leaky' nature of bodies (Michalko 2002; Shildrick 1997).

Sexual bodies on public display

In a society where disabled people are too often constituted as 'genderless, asexual undesirables' (Clare 2015: 130), having sex, and foregrounding sexuality, becomes a resistant act. Lisa and Freddie each have a child, while Richard has three. Warren tells lots of people he is gay, and Joshua is openly bisexual. *What is the message here?* Disabled people fuck, and think of fucking, too.[1] In effect, Lisa, Freddie, Richard, Warren, and Joshua are cripping pervasive ableist attitudes about normative sex and reproduction, family, and upbringing.

Shildrick (2007) has highlighted how disabled people are constantly desexualised by others throughout their lives, whether it be through the exclusion of sexual education classes, close monitoring of 'inappropriate' behaviour, unwelcome or inaccessible sexual health facilities, the infantilisation of disabled people as incapable of making sexual choices, or the belief that disabled sex is disgusting. Many disabled people, much like queer and racial minorities, are also subjected to the idea that they should not—or cannot—contribute to the growth of the human population. Under this view, dominant tropes around sterilisation and eugenics posit that 'faulty genes' should not be reproduced (Siebers 2008). Disabled people who 'flaunt' their sexuality are thus resisting the disavowal of disabled sexual subjectivities, cripping ableist norms about sexual practice, and resisting abjection. Yet moments of resistance sometimes involve more than the disruptive presence of an individual body. They also involve intersubjective and everyday moments of interaction in response to practices of abjection.

Intersubjective encounters

While Amal resisted her school bullying by abandoning her 'friends' who were tormenting her, Joshua sometimes responded to his bullies with physical violence. If Amal does not like some people on the train she will seek assistance from a public transport officer, yet Lisa confronts people and uses crip humour to disarm people's anger that her wheelchair takes up too much space ('OK, would you like me to get my tie ropes out of the bottom of my chair and start tying myself to the roof?'). While Emma has no visible physical differences, she sometimes asks for a ramp when disembarking from a train—distorting onlooker's notions and meanings of (physical) disability/difference (see Fitzgerald and Paterson 1995; Mills 2017). When Jake goes on work placements, telling his new boss about his disability is one of the first things he does. Peter does not talk to his brother any more after he tried to sell Peter's house, and Richard chooses whether to respond when he catches people staring at him. Warren went to the police station to report his sexual assault, and in a more extreme example, Clifton confronted his father as he was dying, telling him that he was angry and hated him. In each of these intersubjective encounters, Amal, Joshua, Lisa, Emma, Jake, Peter, Richard, Warren, and Clifton have each initiated/responded/resisted differently to different forms of abjection. In a world where almost all of the participants in this research were told to ignore their victimisation, their responses are extraordinary, agentic acts.

These intersubjective responses to abjection foreground the extent to which abjection is socially constituted, embodied, and performed by both abled and disabled subjects. Above I have documented several instances where the participants in this research have resisted their abjection. These instances are not exhaustive, but are intended only to prise open the every-day possibilities in which abjection is, and can be, resisted. In this section, however, I move on to consider how abjection can be resisted as a collective practice. While the participants have experienced abjection as individuals, these experiences are created and imposed through collective social and psychic practices that constitute the disabled subject as abject. McClintock's (1995) account of abjection has illustrated how multiple dimensions overlap at different times and in different places to abjectify disabled bodies.

A small body of literature that articulates possibilities for resisting ableist and disablist practices has emerged in recent years (see Bates, Goodley, and Runswick-Cole 2017; Loja et al. 2017; Runswick-Cole and Goodley 2013, 2015). Despite my admiration for this work, I remain concerned that there tends to be an overemphasis on resistance as an individual practice, and an under-exploration of resistance as a relational and collective practice. My aim in this conclusion is to address this lacuna by de-individualising our responses to abjection and promoting a coalitional relational ethics that mobilises against forms of disabled abjection. Borrowing from Halperin's (2007) observation in Genet's story, those who resist abjection alone may simply be crushed. Consequently, I suggest that it should not be left entirely to individuals to resist their own abjection. Recognising that abjection is a socially produced phenomenon is central to my argument in this book; resistance likewise requires a collective response. The aim of the relational politics I propose is to work performatively against the norms that fail to recognise non-normative bodies as legitimate and unjustly subject to violence.

Collective action is required in resisting the norms that negate disabled ontologies. If norms become norms through (collective) repetition, then collective action is required to subvert them. Norms, as socially constituted, 'precede us and act upon us', and oblige us to re/produce them. And yet, in their enactment 'something may go awry' (Butler 2015: 31). When this occurs, 'some weakness of the norm is revealed', and 'another desire starts to govern, and forms of resistance develop, something new occurs, [and] not previously what was planned' (Butler 2015: 31). When a norm comes to someone, it comes from someone/something else. For example, someone is constituted as disabled because other people are constituted *as such*. Given the power of norms, in order for a norm to be relaxed, resisted or supplanted, collective action that works to enable non-normative bodies and standards to be more possible and liveable is required.

Moving to collective practices of resistance

In trying to resist abjection as a collective practice, my thinking turns to possibilities for collective action. But what might this look like, and how might it work? At this point in a book, a series of recommendations is conventional. *Do this or that. Write this training program. Increase education about this issue.* I resist that temptation to reproduce the idea that I have *the answer*. However, I do want to switch registers slightly and examine ableism, in order to prise open some small ways in which ableism, and in turn, abjection, can be resisted in general terms. This aligns with my project, from above, to posit a collective response to resist abjection, and to destabilise and renegotiate the terms by which disabled people are defined according to regulatory norms. Just as queer theory critiques heteronormativity (see Berlant and Warner 1998; Warner 1993, 1999, for examples), I want to provide a crip critique of ableism and compulsory abledness. I take Goodley's (2017) point that there can be no critical disability studies without political commitment, and I work to shift the gaze (Campbell 2009) away from disabled people and on to ableism in order to highlight some of the ways in which norms might be relaxed, resisted, broken, supplanted, and/or remade.

Activism/advocacy

Nearly all of the participants in this research are involved in the self-advocacy movement, and this is one example of collective resistance. Yet I might suggest, respectfully, an addition to their focus. The self-advocacy movement is largely focussed on fighting for the rights of disabled people, and while this is admirable, necessary, and worthwhile, it might be equally justifiable to advocate for non-normative difference and against ableism. As it stands, one critique of the prevailing self-advocacy approach is that there is too much emphasis on minimising disability, overcoming disability, and showing 'how human' disabled people are and can be (the 'people first' approach comes to mind) (Titchkosky 2007). Instead, I propose—if I can be so brash—the self-advocacy movement adopts vehement critiques of ableism, and puts forth their differences. Such approaches might work to provoke abled people to confront their own precariousness and ableism.

The 'normal body' needs to be exposed as a fiction; Davis (1995: xii) writes that the aim should be 'to help "normal" people see the quotation marks around their state'. Bodies are imperfect, changeable, and unruly, and this needs to be foregrounded to abled people. The disabled body should also be exposed as having experiences, capacities, and positions that are unavailable to abled people:

[n]ot only do physically disabled people[2] have experiences, which are not available to the able-bodied, they are in a better position to transcend cultural mythologies about the body, because they *cannot* do things that the able-bodied feel they *must* do in order to be happy, 'normal' and sane.

(Wendell 1992: 77)

In this example, the practices that Wendell (1992) describes expose the precariousness of bodies, and in effect, crips them. Putting disabledness on show—which many of the participants in this research have encountered—works to crip the environment and highlight the ableist practices with which people engage.

Foregrounding the sexual practices of disabled people is another example that works to expose differences that are unavailable, or not yet realisable, to abled people. Disabled people and abled people may have very different notions of what erogenous zones are, what they do, and where they are (Siebers 2008). Wilensky (2001: np) documents her heightened sensitivity:

[b]ecause I am so sensitive to touch, so acutely aware of a breeze on my neck, a ring on my finger, the rib of a sock pressing into my ankle, when I choose to participate in sexual contact, my unusually heightened physicality works for and not against me.

Disabled people experience sex in very similar and very different ways to each other and abled people. Disabled people open spaces of possibility that many abled people may not have imagined, flagging possibilities for alternative sexual techniques, experimentations, and diversities. Highlighting the 'mythical norm' (Lorde 1984: 116) to abled people and the ways in which disabled bodies can be exceptional and extraordinary (Garland Thomson 1996, 1997)—rather than deficient and lacking—exposes their own abled precariousness, and spaces of possibility open to dis/abled lives.

Education

Following Goodley (2014), I suggest it might also be useful to educate abled and ableist people about the ableism and abjection they wrongfully re-instantiate and perpetuate. While there are endless articles, instructions, and pamphlets available that illustrate how abled people should communicate with disabled people, what if we also provided information about how disabled people and their allies should engage with the ableist and disablist subject? Goodley (2014: 134) creates the name of a possible pamphlet title: *Dis/ability Etiquette: Tips on Interacting with Normal People*. Goodley's (2014) crip parody appropriately shifts the gaze away from disabled people and on to ableism.

Ball's (2002) article, 'Who'd Fuck an Ableist?', also points to the inverted focus from disability to ableism, and highlights how it is not disabled people who have 'problems', but ableist people who are problematic with their messy abjectifying behaviours. Rather than help 'normal people' communicate with disabled people, disabled people and their allies should also be trained about how to deal with the 'psychopathology of the normals' (Goodley 2014: 117) and their obsession with normativity. These approaches might adequately stoke abled people's ontological insecurities, and force them to (re)question their own ableist attitudes. Indeed, is this book perhaps what Goodley (2014) (maybe) had in mind?

Celebration and display

Rather than re-instantiate discourses of cure, rehabilitation, and therapy for disabled people, let disabled people trouble normative standards instilled in our culture by celebrating and displaying their differences. Much like many of the participants in this research, and whether deliberate or not, abnormality can be the basis for a form of counterculture activism; one that can reconfigure the normative meanings of abnormality. For example, the 'disruptive child' could become the 'productive child', the 'wheelchair-bound', the 'human-machine hybrid', and the 'intellectually disabled', the 'distribution of intelligence' (Goodley 2017). Putting dis/ability on display can disrupt notions of what it means to be human, and disrupts normal people's normative ableist beliefs. Celebrating abnormality works to disrupt the integrity of normality.

The freak show, as it is conventionally understood, is one example of the ways in which disabled people have historically been constituted as objects of entertainment. During their peak in popularity in the late nineteenth and early twentieth century, disabled people were bought, sold, and traded between managers, and exploited for profit based on their disability (Clare 2015; Gerber 1996). Under this view, disabled people had no/little agency, and they were used for the enjoyment of abled people. Another view, which I am more sympathetic to, is that the freak shows served to expose to abled people their own precariousness and corporeal fragility (Bogdan 1988; Garland Thomson 1997).

Some researchers have also suggested that 'freaks' were not passive victims subjected to exploitation, but in many cases possessed the agency to make willing decisions, perform for others, and earn an income (Bogdan 1988; Clare 2015). During the period of freak shows, many abled people also sought to create/exhibit disability, such as 'freaks' growing beards, getting tattoos, hiding their arms to create the impression that they were amputees, pretending to be a conjoined twin, and so on (Bogdan 1988). These behaviours and practices highlight the performative nature of identity and non-normative bodies, illuminate the 'leakiness' of bodies (Shildrick 1997), and confront ableist people with their own ableism. Recognising that the 'freak show is [not] all that dead', Clare (2015: 100) points out that other iterations and practices have now replaced the traditional freak show, and that flagging and flaunting non-normative identities in public settings expose ableist thoughts and practices. The re-emergence of the freak show and the growth of disabled (solo autobiographical) performance pieces (see Fernández and Conejo 2017; Sandahl 2003) points to the rise of such practices.

Final thoughts

Above I have worked through some ideas about how abjection can be resisted. As I have documented in this and the 'Social Abjection and Reappropriation' chapter, the cultural terms by which we live are changeable. Dis/ability can be thought otherwise, and normative standards subverted. Abjection can also be resisted or reclaimed by throwing it back in ableist faces, returning the stare, and accepting the hail. Yet I have emphasised a collective relational ethics is required to recast the dimensions of abjection as dimensions as resistance. Lisa, Roger, Deb, Jake, Anne-Marie, Amal, Emma, Freddie, Joshua, Peter, Warren, Richard, and Clifton cannot do it on their own. Collective effort is required, as it is only through exposing everyone's precariousness that we can generate actions that create interdependence, promote difference, and a shared empathy. I have highlighted spaces where disabled people can live the transcendence I have described, speak back and return the gaze, renegotiate or recast the terms by which they are defined, and, perhaps most importantly, live crip.

Notes

1 Yet I also do not want to foreclose the idea that there is a legitimate group of disabled people, like all people, who do identify as asexual (see Kim 2011).
2 I think this applies to all forms of disability, not just physically disabled people.

References

Ball, KF 2002, 'Who'd Fuck an Ableist?', *Disability Studies Quarterly*, 22(4): 166–172.
Barad, K 2007, *Meeting the Universe Halfway: Quantum Physics and the Entanglement of Matter and Meaning*, Duke University Press, Durham and London.
Bates, K, Goodley, D, and Runswick-Cole, K 2017, 'Precarious Lives and Resistant Possibilities: The Labour of People with Learning Disabilities in Times of Austerity', *Disability & Society*, 32(2): 160–175.
Berlant, L and Warner, M 1998, 'Sex in Public', *Critical Inquiry*, 24(2): 547–566.
Bogdan, R 1988, *Freak Show: Presenting Human Oddities for Amusement and Profit*, The University of Chicago Press, Chicago and London.

Butler, J 2009, 'Performativity, Precarity and Sexual Politics', *Revista De Antropología Iberoamericana*, 4(3): i–xiii.

Butler, J 2015, *Notes toward a Performative Theory of Assembly*, Harvard University Press, Cambridge, MA.

Campbell, FK 2009, *Contours of Ableism: The Production of Disability and Abledness*, Palgrave Macmillan, London and New York.

Clare, E 2015, *Exile and Pride: Disability, Queerness, and Liberation*, 16th anniversary edition, Duke University Press, Durham and London.

Davis, LJ 1995, *Enforcing Normalcy: Disability, Deafness, and the Body*, Verso, London and New York.

Fernández, AG and Conejo, MA 2017, 'Playing Crip: The Politics of Disabled Artists' Performances in Spain', *Research in Drama Education: The Journal of Applied Theatre and Performance*, 22(3): 345–351.

Fitzgerald, MH and Paterson, KA 1995, 'The Hidden Disability Dilemma for the Preservation of Self', *Journal of Occupational Science*, 2(1): 13–21.

Garland Thomson, R 1996, 'Introduction: From Wonder to Error—A Genealogy of Freak Discourse in Modernity', in *Freakery: Cultural Spectacles of the Extraordinary Body*, edited by R Garland Thomson, New York University Press, New York and London, pp. 1–19.

Garland Thomson, R 1997, *Extraordinary Bodies: Figuring Physical Disability in American* Culture *and Literature*, Columbia University Press, New York.

Garland-Thomson, R 2009, *Staring: How We Look*, Oxford University Press, New York.

Gerber, DA 1996, 'The "Careers" of People Exhibited in Freak Shows: The Problem of Volition and Valorization', in *Freakery: Cultural Spectacles of the Extraordinary Body*, edited by R Garland Thomson, New York University Press, New York and London, pp. 38–54.

Goodley, D 2014, *Dis/ability Studies: Theorising Disablism and Ableism*, Routledge, London and New York.

Goodley, D 2017, *Disability Studies: An Interdisciplinary Introduction*, 2nd edition, SAGE, London.

Halperin, DM 2007, *What Do Gay Men Want? An Essay on Sex, Risk, and Subjectivity*, The University of Michigan Press, Ann Arbor, MI.

Kim, E 2011, 'Asexuality in Disability Narratives', *Sexualities*, 14(4): 479–493.

Kristeva, J 1982, *Powers of Horror: An Essay on Abjection*, translated by LS Roudiez, Columbia University Press, New York.

Loja, E, Costa, ME, Hughes, B, and Menezes, I 2017, 'Disability, Embodiment and Ableism: Stories of Resistance', *Disability & Society*, 28(2): 190–203.

Lorde, A 1984, *Sister Outsider: Essays and Speeches by Audre Lorde*, The Crossing Press, Freedom, CA.

McClintock, A 1995, *Imperial Leather: Race, Gender and Sexuality in the Colonial Contest*, Routledge, New York and London.

McRuer, R 2006, *Crip Theory: Cultural Signs of Queerness and Disability*, New York University Press, New York and London.

Meijer, IC and Prins, B (with J Butler) 1998, 'How Bodies Come to Matter: An Interview with Judith Butler', *Signs: Journal of Women in Culture and Society*, 23(2): 275–286.

Michalko, R 1999, *The Two-In-One: Walking with Smokie, Walking with Blindness*, Temple University Press, Philadelphia, PA.

Michalko, R 2002, *The Difference that Disability Makes*, Temple University Press, Philadelphia, PA.

Mills, C 2015, 'Undoing Ethics: Butler on Precarity, Opacity and Responsibility', in *Butler and Ethics*, edited by M Lloyd, Edinburgh University Press, Edinburgh, pp. 41–64.

Mills, ML 2017, 'Invisible Disabilities, Visible Service Dogs: The Discrimination of Service Dog Handlers', *Disability & Society*, 32(5): 635–656.

Morris, J 1991, *Pride against Prejudice: A Personal Politics of Disability*, Women's Press, London.

Reeve, D 2002, 'Negotiating Psycho-emotional Dimensions of Disability and Their Influence on Identity Constructions', *Disability & Society*, 17(5): 493–508.

Runswick-Cole, K and Goodley, D 2013, 'Resilience: A Disability Studies and Community Psychology Approach', *Social and Personality Psychology Compass*, 7(2): 67–78.

Runswick-Cole, K and Goodley, D 2015, 'Disability, Austerity and Cruel Optimism in Big Society: Resistance and "The Disability Commons"', *Canadian Journal of Disability Studies*, 4(2): 162–186.

Sandahl, C 2003, 'Queering the Crip or Cripping the Queer? Intersections of Queer and Crip Identities in Solo Autobiographical Performance', *GLQ: A Journal of Lesbian and Gay Studies*, 9(1–2): 25–56.

Shildrick, M 1997, *Leaky Bodies and Boundaries: Feminism, Postmodernism and Bio-(ethics)*, Routledge, London and New York.

Shildrick, M 2007, 'Contested Pleasures: The Sociopolitical Economy of Disability and Sexuality', *Sexuality Research & Social Policy*, 4(1): 53–66.

Siebers, T 2008, *Disability Theory*, The University of Michigan Press, Ann Arbor, MI.

Swain, J, Heyman, B, and Gillman, M 1998, 'Public Research, Private Concerns: Ethical Issues in the Use of Open-ended Interviews with People Who Have Learning Difficulties', *Disability & Society*, 13(1): 21–36.

Titchkosky, T 2007, *Reading and Writing Disability Differently: The Textured Life of Embodiment*, University of Toronto Press, Toronto.

Warner, M (ed.) 1993, *Fear of a Queer Planet: Queer Politics and Social Theory*, University of Minnesota Press, Minneapolis and London.

Warner, M 1999, *The Trouble with Normal: Sex, Politics, and the Ethics of Queer Life*, Harvard University Press, Cambridge, MA.

Wendell, S 1992, 'Toward a Feminist Theory of Disability', in *Feminist Perspectives in Medical Ethics*, edited by HB Holmes and LM Purdy, Indiana University Press, Bloomington and Indianapolis, pp. 63–81.

Wilensky, A 2001, 'The Skin I'm In', *Nerve*, 24 October, accessed online 9 February 2017, web.archive.org/web/20011103041347/www.nerve.com/PersonalEssays/Wilensky/skin/

Appendix
Research method(ology)

The qualitative research drawn on in this book began in May 2015 and ended in April 2016, and it was done as part of doctoral work completed in the School of Social Sciences and Psychology at Western Sydney University. Participants were recruited from three different disability organisations, and each participant was asked to recount various aspects of their life and experiences. Below I outline several details that are required to fully understand the life history narratives, their presentation in the book, and my approach to the research data.

The interviews

All interviews, except one, took place at the offices of the disability organisations or self-advocacy groups. I made this decision because it was the location each participant was familiar with, and there were other people, namely support workers, who were in close proximity to each interview should the participant request their presence/assistance. The sole interview that did not occur at these locations was with Jake; instead, this interview was held in a private room on university campus. At the start of each interview, I went through the participant information sheet and consent form, and this took varying lengths of time depending on the participants' ability to comprehend the material and my own ability to communicate in an appropriate way. For the most part, the consent process took about ten minutes, but sometimes it took up to twenty minutes. For some participants I introduced red and yellow signs; the red sign said 'Stop Interview', while the yellow sign said 'Next Question'. They were invited to hold up whichever sign whenever they desired. I did this for a couple of reasons. In illuminating experiences of abjection, I became very cognisant of trying not to abjectify the participants. As Swain, Heyman, and Gillman (1998: 22) speculate, 'research that gives voice to the experiences of abuse can itself be abusive', and I was trying to come up with strategies that did not commit acts of (symbolic) violence against the participants. Also, as someone who appreciates multiple and unstable notions of meaning and communication, I tried to think of various ways that enabled the participants to communicate, rather than remove their agency or commit violence/abjection against them in an interview space. For some people, showing a sign is easier than verbally communicating, and I wanted to signify that alternative methods could be employed to halt interviews or lines of questioning. As an example, some may consider the act of a participant falling asleep as a sign of tiredness, yet it may in fact represent a strategic choice by the participant to illustrate they are removing their consent, or do not appreciate a certain line of questioning (see Rodgers 1999). I can recall only one circumstance when the 'Next Question' sign was used. Overall, each interview was conducted in a mutually respectful manner.

Working with the transcripts

A Foucauldian-inspired analysis of discourse guided my examination of the thirteen life histories I conducted. In this section I briefly illustrate how the data were analysed using this approach. Some scholars such as Parker (1992), Kendall and Wickham (1999), Arribas-Ayllon and Walkerdine (2008), and Willig (2003) have identified various stages and steps when performing this type of analysis. Rather than adopt any single approach over another, I was informed by, and borrowed from, each in different ways. It should be highlighted that I did not complete these steps sequentially, nor do I consider these steps mutually exclusive. The summary I provide below describes what is ultimately a 'messy' (Law 2004) and 'intuitive' (Hollway 1989) process, given there are no set rules for conducting a Foucauldian-inspired analysis of discourse (Arribas-Ayllon and Walkerdine 2008).

Yet before outlining how I worked with the transcripts, I should restate how Foucault's (1972, 1978, 1980) notions of discourse, discursive practices, and the regulation of the subject informed my analysis. Discourse, according to Foucault (1972), refers to the meanings, statements, and representations that congeal to create a particular version of 'reality', and power is central to the ways in which discourses function and are constituted. Recognising that power is productive and entwined with knowledge (1978), Foucault (1980: 93) suggests,

> [i]n a society such as ours, but basically in any society, there are manifold relations of power which permeate, characterise and constitute the social body, and these relations of power cannot themselves be established, consolidated nor implemented without the production, accumulation, circulation and functioning of discourse.

For Foucault, discourse governs the ways in which topics are discussed (through power), and the ways in which subjects are constituted and regulated. Some of the aims of a Foucauldian-inspired analysis of discourse are to consider the ways in which discourses influence topics that are discussed, transmit and produce power, and regulate subjects. Importantly, it also helps to identify spaces in which discourses can be challenged and transformed. I work with Foucault's (1972, 1978, 1980) notion of discourse and discursive practices in this project to consider the discourses (not) drawn upon by the thirteen participants, how these discourses constitute and regulate them, and speculate about their meanings and social implications.

At the time of analysis, I approached this study with the intention of theorising experiences of violence as abjection. In my preliminary analysis, then, I moved through each transcript looking for experiences of violence and the ways in which the participants constructed these experiences. My conceptualisation of violence extended beyond conventional understandings; in addition to physical acts, I was looking for experiences of symbolic and normative violence (Butler 1990, 2004), both inflicted upon disabled bodies and by disabled bodies upon themselves. I approached the transcripts with care, patience, and contemplation. I read and re-read, and I used coloured markers to highlight each of the experiences I identified. Each incident was coded and then tabulated according to the type of violence (physical, sexual, verbal, and so on), location (in the home, in public, at school, and so on), relation to the offender (family, friend, known other, stranger, and so on), and so on. I also examined and coded their experiences towards violence, such as what they did, who they told, and how they felt about it.

But I was not solely looking at violence. As I discussed in the opening chapter, my thinking had also moved to questions of subjectivity, and inherent to the nature of life histories, I was focussed on their narratives. In later examinations of the transcripts, I became preoccupied with *who the participants were*. I started to consider the narratives of each individual participant, looking at the particularities of their lives. One by one, I mapped out a life history of each participant: where they grew up; what their families were like; what experiences they had and how they felt about them; their dreams, frustrations, hopes, disappointments; and so on. I looked at whatever they told me, and examined the inclusions and omissions, depth and breadth, similarities and points of departure. I read the transcripts for their plot, their voice ('I'; but also when the 'I' was displaced), their relationships, and their position within broader social and cultural forces (see Mauthner and Doucet 1998). I became preoccupied with the discourses they drew upon, the subject positions they occupied, and I speculated about their social implications.

In subsequent readings and analyses I became concerned with re-theorising their experiences of violence as abjection, predominately using Kristeva (1982), Butler (1993, in Meijer and Prins 1998), and McClintock's (1995) frameworks. Incorporating their life experiences and re-theorising violence as abjection, I wrote out each individual life history for the thirteen participants. I whittled down 500,000 words of transcript to about 50,000 words of life histories. Inevitably, working out how to structure these life histories within this book—where word limits and convention are highly regulated—became difficult to manage. In hindsight, I conducted too many life histories; perhaps quantitative thinking slipped into my qualitative research. However, I also do not want to leave the impression that I regret meeting these participants and learning about their lives.

I took considerable time and contemplation when devising an adequate book structure. It would have been pragmatic to focus on only a few life histories, and choose to focus on only the most relevant to my theorising. Yet I was cognisant that invisibilising some participants' contributions in this research would be a form of symbolic violence (see Bourdieu 1991; Butler 1997)[1] and abjection, and I wanted to avoid this as much as possible.[2] To omit participants' contributions entirely from this book would send the message that their stories are not worth hearing, or that they should not have bothered participating in project in the first place. I did not want their contributions to go to waste in this book. Thinking through these issues, the aims of this research shifted towards building a psychic and social account of abjection and working with McClintock's (1995) framework for identifying multiple dimensions of abjection. Given these shifting aims, each of the chapters in this book serves a slightly different purpose, and as I identify below, I approached each of the participants' narratives in slightly different ways depending on the specific and shifting foci of my analyses.

In the first two 'results' chapters, I used McClintock's (1995) framework to explore Deb and Roger's life histories and expose the multi-dimensional forms of abjection in their lives. I did this to illuminate the compounding, reiterative, and distributed nature of abjection, and to show how exterior social discourses and practices shape Deb and Roger's experiences of abjection. Following this, I introduced the biographies of the other eleven participants in order to contextualise their accounts before considering, in chapter six, the interior or psychic dimensions of abjection. Specifically, I exposed how many of the participants self-abjected through pathologising and disavowing their disabled subjectivities. I then worked with Anne-Marie's life history narrative in chapter seven to expose the simultaneously social and psychic, individual and collective forms of abjection. Importantly, however, in trying to open spaces of possibility in which abjection can be resisted, I foregrounded moments in Anne-Marie's narrative where she had resisted her own abjection.

Notes

1 I follow Bourdieu's (1991) and Butler's (1997) understandings that symbolic violence is a form of violence that is inflicted upon bodies without the knowledge, feeling, or recognition that violence is being committed.
2 After all, I have already committed symbolic violence by re-working their narratives, including and excluding, prioritising and de-prioritising parts of their stories for my own purposes.

References

Arribas-Ayllon, M and Walkerdine, V 2008, 'Foucauldian Discourse Analysis', in *The SAGE Handbook of Qualitative Research in Psychology*, edited by C Willig and W Stainton-Rogers, SAGE Publications, London, pp. 91–108.

Bourdieu, P 1991, *Language and Symbolic Power*, Harvard University Press, Cambridge, MA.

Butler, J 1990, *Gender Trouble: Feminism and the Subversion of Identity*, Routledge, New York and London.

Butler, J 1993, *Bodies that Matter: On the Discursive Limits of 'Sex'*, Routledge, New York and London.

Butler, J 1997, *Excitable Speech: A Politics of the Performative*, Routledge, New York and London.

Butler, J 2004, *Precarious Life: The Powers of Mourning and Violence*, Verso, London and New York.

Foucault, M 1972, *Archaeology of Knowledge*, translated by A.M Sheridan Smith, Routledge, London.

Foucault, M 1978, *The History of Sexuality, Vol. I: An Introduction*, translated by Robert Hurley, Pantheon Books, New York.

Foucault, M 1980, 'Two Lectures', in *Power/Knowledge: Selected Interviews and Other Writings, 1972–1977*, edited by C Gordon, Harvester Press Ltd, Sussex, pp. 78–108.

Hollway, W 1989, *Subjectivity and Method in Psychology: Gender, Meaning and Science*, SAGE Publications, London.

Kendall, G and Wickham, G 1999, *Using Foucault's Methods*, SAGE Publications, London.

Kristeva, J 1982, *Powers of Horror: An Essay on Abjection*, translated by LS Roudiez, Columbia University Press, New York.

Law, J 2004, *After Method: Mess in Social Science Research*, Routledge, New York.

Mauthner, N and Doucet, A 1998, 'Reflections on a Voice-centred Relational Method: Analysing Maternal and Domestic Voices', in *Feminist Dilemmas in Qualitative Research: Public Knowledge and Private Lives*, edited by J Ribbens and R Edwards, SAGE Publications, London, pp. 119–146.

McClintock, A 1995, *Imperial Leather: Race, Gender and Sexuality in the Colonial Contest*, Routledge, New York and London.

Meijer, IC and Prins, B (with J Butler) 1998, 'How Bodies Come to Matter: An Interview with Judith Butler', *Signs: Journal of Women in Culture and Society*, 23(2): 275–286.

Parker, I 1992, *Discourse Dynamics: Critical Analysis for Social and Individual Psychology*, Routledge, London and New York.

Rodgers, J 1999, 'Trying to Get It Right: Undertaking Research Involving People with Learning Difficulties', *Disability & Society*, 14(4): 421–433.

Swain, J, Heyman, B, and Gillman, M 1998, 'Public Research, Private Concerns: Ethical Issues in the Use of Open-Ended Interviews with People Who Have Learning Difficulties', *Disability & Society*, 13(1): 21–36.

Willig, C 2003, 'Discourse Analysis', in *Qualitative Psychology: A Practical Guide to Research Methods*, edited by JA Smith, SAGE Publications, London, pp. 159–183.

Index

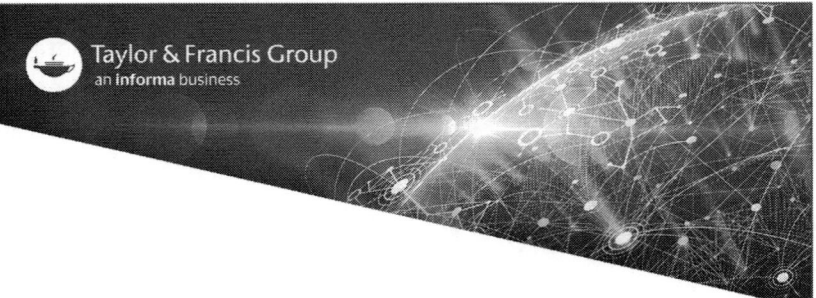
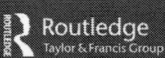
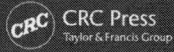